Finding Heroes:

The Search for Columbia's Astronauts

Byron Starr

LIAISON PRESS

VANCOUVER · BRITISH COLUMBIA · CANADA

Finding Heroes: The Search for Columbia's Astronauts

by Byron Starr

Published by Liaison Press, an imprint of Creative Guy Publishing.
www.liaisonpress.com
www.creativeguypublishing.com
CGP-4009
ISBN 1-894953-41-X
October 2006
Trade edition

Library and Archives Canada Cataloguing in Publication
Starr, Byron, 1972-
Finding heroes : the search for Columbia's astronauts / Byron Starr.
ISBN 1-894953-41-X
ISBN 1-894953-42-8 (bound)
ISBN 1-894953-43-6 (ebook)
1. Columbia (Spacecraft)--Accidents. 2. Volunteer workers in search and rescue operations--Texas--Sabine County. 3. Starr, Byron, 1972-.
I. Title.
HV551.4.T4S73 2006 362.12'492 C2006-903848-1

Finding Heroes:

The Search for Columbia's Astronauts

Byron Starr

L I A I S O N   P R E S S
VANCOUVER·BRITISH COLUMBIA·CANADA

In Memory of Bernice Nethery and Geraldine Reeves.

and

In Honor of Kathleen White

Table of Contents:

Acknowledgements..1

Forward..3

1. Out of the Clear Morning Sky..5

2. Reaction and Response..7

3. Bringing it Together..17

4. Setting Protocol..25

5. Into the Woods..35

6. With Dignity and Respect...49

7. The Media...63

8. The Nose Cone and the Space Monkeys..............................69

9. Walking The Woods..77

10. The Third Day's Recoveries..81

11. Logistics and Communication..89

12. Medical Response...95

13. Lending a Hand...101

14. Bronson's Dogs...107

15. The Fourth Day's Recoveries...111

16. Trudging Through the Cold Rain.....................................121

17. A Privilege...129

18. Moving the Nose Cone...133

19. The Air Search..137

20. Reporting on Sabine County...145

21. On and Below Toledo Bend...151

22. Uncooperative Weather..159

23. The Expanding Operation...167

24. Feeding the Masses..181

25. Back to Work..185

26. The Red Cross..197

27. The Last of the Seven Heroes...203

28. The Memorial Service and Beyond.................................211

Acknowledgements

The following is a list of people who have helped me in one way or another. They are listed in the approximate order in which I contacted them or they contacted me. This list was made from a combination of sketchy notes and even sketchier memory; I apologize if I've left anyone out.

Shelly Starr, John Starr Jr., Fred Raney, Roger McBride, Don Iles, Jason Pearson, Bob Morgan, Laura Krantz, Eric Ruggeri, Megan Bulloch, Pete Allen, Lin and Amy Marcantel, Tony and Jan Alexander, Tracy Lane, Bradley Byley, Linda Campbell, Kim Fox, Tracy Tatom, Charlotte Chance, Sherry Hutto, Wyatt and Ellen Watson, Greg Cohrs, Marc Griffin, Steve Mills, Raymond Lofton, Jamie Brasher, Pat Oden, Jamie Williams, Chip Robberson, Duane Husband, Steve Dougharty, Billy Rowles, Nathan Ener, Kathy Lane, Stanley Christopher, David and Rhonda Whitmire, Don Rodriguez, Billy Ted Smith, Mark Allen, Lisa Owens, Steve Miller, Joe Simmons, Murray Kilgore, Charlie Creech, Fred Salinas, Gay Ippolitto, Don Eddings, Jack Leath, Cookie Cryer, Ardath Mayhar, Todd Parrish, Felix Holmes, Jerry Kidd, Butch and Jalain Andrews, John Whitten, Mike Defee, Janie Peveto Johnson, Mary Beth Grey, Hank Lavine, Pat Payne, Laverne Harris, Brenda Crow, Herbert and Amber Welch, Bill and Kathy Collier, Steve and Doris Arney, Kathleen White, Jim Steele, Ginger Ellis, Marsha Cooper.

Forward

This is the story of how various federal, state, and local agencies and organizations, first responders and a community of volunteers worked together with one goal in mind—to bring Columbia's heroes home to their families. In this search for heroes, we found heroes among ourselves, from the tireless volunteers walking the search line, to the organizers in the Incident Command Center. While my own greatest accomplishment might be summed up as an ability to stay out of the way and occasionally help carry a stretcher, I feel fortunate to have worked with outstanding people.

It is not the intention of this book to place any one person or organization in higher standing than another—no one person or organization could have accomplished what we, as a team, accomplished. However, these people have been used as representatives of everyone involved. I should also mention that, while the effort in Sabine County, Texas, was unique in that all seven astronauts were recovered in the area, one should keep in mind that likeminded first responders and volunteers were diligently combing the woods all up and down Columbia's flight path. Unless otherwise noted, all of the towns and cities named are in Texas.

Portions of this book deal directly with the recovery of Columbia's astronauts. However, out of respect for the astronauts and their family I have tried to treat my accounts of the recoveries with the same dignity we showed them during the operation.

1

Out of the Clear Morning Sky

A T FIRST there was a sound not unlike deep, rolling thunder in the distance. Those of us who were already awake on that beautiful Saturday morning thought it odd to hear this on such a clear morning, but no one could have imagined what this distant sound heralded.

As the sound continued to grow in volume it became apparent that this was not ordinary thunder. It was less of a natural roll and more like an irregular series of booms. Within seconds this sound had increased to the point that it sounded more like a rapid series of muffled explosions.

By this time, those of us who were still in bed were waking to what many thought was a nightmare. Window frames rattled, pictures fell from walls, and still the horrible sound grew louder. As we began to realize that this nightmare was really happening, many panicked minds reached out, grasping the most terrible possibilities they could imagine, everything from pipeline explosions to nuclear war and even Armageddon. In hindsight it's easy to laugh off such wild reactions, but, at the time, our fears were very real. And, unlike real nightmares, where we jerk awake at the instant the terror grips us, this nightmare kept on coming. The sound grew to such a crescendo that the walls of our houses began to shake. And some even had the added horror of opening their windows to see jagged pieces of twisted metal raining from the sky.

Mercifully, after several long minutes the booms reached their peak and began to taper off. Fear lingered, but panic began to melt away. Typical of people in any rural area, most of us reached for the phone and began calling friends and family to make sure everyone was okay and to see if anyone knew what had happened. A few of us realized that the hellish thunder had sounded, and even felt, like a series of sonic booms, but no one had a clue what had really happened until they turned on their televisions.

At that time the rest of the world was holding their breath as it had just become known that Houston had lost contact with the Space Shuttle Columbia. Those of us along the shuttle's path put two and two together and realized that the shuttle, along with her seven brave crewmembers, had been lost.

Fear changed to sorrow, and this sorrow quickly turned to determination. Over the next few days this determination spread like a fever through the locals and the volunteers and emergency response workers who would be arriving in droves. It was this determination that found its way into the hearts of everyone, from the common volunteer on the search line to the officials of the dozens of state, federal, and local organizations that oversaw the operation. It was this determination that overcame every difficulty imaginable in some of the harshest terrain in the country to not just recover of the vast majority of the shuttle itself, but also to recover of all seven of Columbia's crew within the first eleven days of the operation.

2

Reaction and Response

IN A RURAL sheriff's department, like the one in Sabine County, the 911 emergency phone is treated with great respect. It rarely rang, but when it did, something big was happening.

Amy Marcantel and Wyatt Watson were working the dispatch office at the Blan Greer Law Enforcement Center on the morning of February 1, 2003. The dispatcher, Amy usually handled the phones while Wyatt, the jailor, took care of the inmates. However it was a bit of an ongoing joke between the two of them that the 911 phone never rang until Amy was out of the office. As it turned out, Amy had just stepped out for a cigarette break at eight o'clock that morning. Wyatt was in the dispatch office talking with Royce Warr, who oversaw the county's community service program, when a distant rumbling began. This rumbling crescendoed until the walls of the heavy concrete jail were shaking. As the strange, loud tremor faded, Wyatt turned to Royce and said, "We're going to know what that was, real quick."

No sooner had the words come out of his mouth than the 911 phone rang.

The caller identified himself and said he was from Bronson, which is a small community located ten miles west of Hemphill. "Things are falling all around my house," the man said. "I think an airliner has crashed or something."

An airliner crash or disintegrating and falling from the sky was the first thing that had crossed Wyatt's mind as well. He took down the man's address and told him a deputy would be on the way as soon as possible. Before Wyatt could get off the line, much less get to the radio, one of the 911 backup lines started ringing.

The second call was a lady who practically shouted, "What was that?"

"Ma'am, I think we have an aircraft down or going down in the area. I really don't have any more information at this time," Wyatt politely replied, hurrying the lady off the phone so he could catch another incoming call.

Amy darted back into the dispatcher's office and caught one of several calls coming in. By this time all five of the emergency lines were lit up, as were all five of the regular lines.

A few minutes after the pandemonium had begun, one of the callers informed Wyatt that Houston had lost contact with the space shuttle. Wyatt turned to the TV resting on a high shelf in the dispatcher's office. The volume was low, but the picture on the screen showed Mission Control in Houston. The ticker tape running along the bottom of the screen gave enough information for Wyatt to realize what had happened.

There was no time for shock or disbelief, however, as hundreds of calls reporting debris, and even more calls from people who simply wanted answers, continued to pour into the sheriff's department. For the first few hours, all ten lines were constantly lit up, which, in effect, added fuel to the fire. The locals realized how rare a 911 call was in the county, so when they called and found all the lines tied up, they knew something terrible must have happened. People frantically redialed the number until they could get through.

Although Sheriff Tom Maddox was just down the hall in his office, with the phones still ringing off the walls and the dispatch radio to worry about, getting word to him was easier said than done. While Wyatt temporarily manned all the phone lines and the radio, Amy sprinted out the door and down the hall to the sheriff's office. She burst in the door and told the sheriff what was happening; then she turned and ran back to the dispatcher's office. Tom immediately left his office and started for Bronson.

During the first couple of hours, Amy and Wyatt did all they could to keep at least one line open. They didn't want someone to try to call in a local emergency, like a house fire or a vehicle accident, and find all the lines tied up. Some of the calls were much like the second of the day—a simple, "What was that?" Other calls were reporting that they had witnessed three large objects with a long white vapor trail passing overhead in the clear blue sky. And quite a few calls, especially those coming in from the Bronson area, were actually reporting falling debris. With everything happening so fast, the information on these first reports was taken as quickly as possible and then set aside until there was enough time and personnel to handle them.

After the first couple of hectic hours, several off-duty dispatchers and other county employees and officials came in to help Amy and Wyatt after, but it was still a madhouse. The calls continued pouring in, almost nonstop, for twelve solid hours.

Not all of the calls were from the locals, however. Almost as soon as the tragedy became known throughout the nation, neighboring police agencies began calling to offer their services. The local volunteer fire departments—and even fire departments from neighboring counties—called to see if there was anything they could do to help. Individual citizens began calling in, asking to lend a hand. Even though the tragedy was less than an hour old, and the recovery operation had yet to begin, volunteers were already offering assistance.

* * *

When the space shuttle Columbia reached Sabine County, she was already in several pieces, some large, some small, most of them still traveling well over the speed of sound. In Dallas, the sound was reported as a pair of distant booms, which is actually normal for a craft the size of the space shuttle—one boom for the nose, another for the tail. However, the residents of Sabine County heard a series of earth shaking booms that were so close together they sounded somewhat like rumbling thunder, yet distinct enough that we knew the sound was nothing nature had produced. Add to this the horror of actually seeing pieces of warped, smoking metal debris falling from the sky and one can understand the panic and confusion that many of the locals felt that morning.

There was a fishing tournament taking place on the Toledo Bend Reservoir that morning. While the sky was clear throughout most of the county, there was still a heavy blanket of fog over the lake. However, a number of witnesses reported seeing debris falling into the water. Some of the fishermen near the southern portion of the lake saw the debris fall all around their boats. The rain of debris was so intense that many of these fishermen actually dove into the bottom of their boats for shelter, while others beached their boats and took shelter on the shore under trees. One particularly panicked fisherman actually dove into the cold water in order to take shelter under his boat.

Literally hundreds of reports of falling debris flooded the Sheriff's Department on the morning of February 1, quickly overwhelming the county's law enforcement assets. Even with the reserve deputies called in, they needed more manpower to respond to the immediate disaster. The Texas Department of Public Safety was contacted; they promised to send troopers as soon as possible. Help was on the way, but for now Sabine County, like the other counties along the shuttle's path, would have to work with what help they had on hand and whatever immediate assistance they could pull in from neighboring counties.

* * *

As soon as Sheriff Billy Rowles of Jasper County received word of falling debris in the northern portion of his county, he contacted the members of the Jasper County Emergency Corps. The Emergency Corps is a volunteer group of uniformed individuals headquartered at the Jasper County Sheriff's Office complex. The group was founded by former Jasper County Sheriff Aubrey E. Cole. They are used primarily to assist local law enforcement in searching for missing children or adults in the woods, securing crime scenes, retrieving sunken boats or automobiles in lakes and rivers, and to help with manning hurricane and forest fire evacuations. Although based in Jasper County and made up of volunteers from the Jasper area, their area of operation often extends beyond the boundaries of the county. In fact, they were quite familiar with Sabine County and the Toledo Bend Reservoir

Billy then contacted a second Jasper based response organization, the Office of Emergency Management: Jasper, Newton and Sabine Counties. This organization is part of the mutual aid and emergency response guidelines that respond to, and help control situations, like tornadoes, tanker truck spills, and hurricane evacuations. Many of the changes that had just taken place with the Homeland Securities Act affected this organization, which would soon have its name changed to the Office of Homeland Security—Jasper, Newton and Sabine Counties. Billy Ted Smith, the organization's Coordinator, was currently several miles away at his job in Beaumont, so Billy Rowels contacted the Assistant Coordinator, Jasper County Fire Chief Jamie Gunter.

Billy and Jamie moved Emergency Management Corp's mobile command post north of Jasper to Brookeland. Listening to the heavy traffic on the radio, it quickly became apparent that the actual path of the debris was north of Jasper County, and Sabine County was in need of assistance. Billy called the Sabine County Sheriff's Office and spoke briefly with Wyatt Watson. Billy asked if they needed any help. Wyatt replied, "We need all the help we can get."

The two Jasper County organizations responded by transferring their command to Hemphill, taking with them their available resources and most of Jasper's county and city law enforcement agencies. As soon as they arrived, Billy and Jamie met with Sabine County Sheriff Tom Maddox, Chief Deputy

Chad Murray, Hemphill Fire Chief D. B. Chance, and Sergeant Tommy Scales of the Texas Department of Public Safety.

Their first priority was dealing with the various reports of debris coming in from throughout the county. The two crucial sites containing a shuttle crewmember and another containing a crew-related item had already been secured by local authorities before the arrival of the Jasper team, but the hundreds of other calls were still overwhelming the fledgling operation's assets. The immediate answer to the lack of manpower was to utilize the local volunteer fire departments. Throughout the day, the local officers would move to the debris sites as they were called in. If the debris proved to be something of lesser importance— tiles, small pieces of metal—the location was documented and the site was marked with police ribbon. If the debris was something of a more sensitive nature—computer instruments, unidentifiable machinery, and fuel tanks—the site was roped off and a volunteer would be left to watch over it. In some cases, volunteers were stationed at the entrance to dirt roads where several debris sites had been reported in order to keep people away until they could all be identified and investigated.

Another major concern addressed in this first meeting was the safety of the public. The county officials had already been warned that some of the debris could be quite hazardous and that the officers needed to keep the public away from the shuttle debris and to avoid contact if at all possible. The Jasper and Hemphill Fire Departments, and the EMC were able to come up with several Geiger counters to help determine if any of the debris was radioactive. These instruments were used throughout the morning until NASA informed the local officials that the counters wouldn't detect what they were looking for because there were no reactors or radioactive experiments on board the space shuttle. NASA stated that the hazard was caused by toxicity, not radioactivity.

The officers and volunteers were told to avoid touching any debris, and to be particularly wary of fuel or storage tanks. They were told what the chemicals looked and smelled like and were given the symptoms to watch for. If contact with one of the chemicals was suspected, they were told to wash thoroughly with soap and water and then proceed immediately to an emergency room.

Throughout the first week of the recovery, rumors would circulate about locals being hospitalized due to contact with these dangerous chemicals. Some of the hospitals in the area did receive emergency room visits from concerned residents who had contacted shuttle debris. The two hospitals in Nacogdoches received around fifty such patients, Palestine Regional Medical Center saw twenty-five patients, and San Augustine Memorial saw four; however, none of these patients showed symptoms of having contacted the toxins.

During that first morning meeting, it was decided that the Law Enforcement Center was too small to serve as a functional command post. The decision was made to set up the Incident Command Post at the Hemphill Volunteer Fire Department's fire hall. This large metal building with its six bays and oblong back meeting room would serve as the command center for the next two weeks of the recovery operation.

* * *

Usually when rumors of a tragedy begin to make their way through the Sabine County grapevine, the funeral home phone rings off the wall. And since I had been so busy answering my own phone before I left for the office, I expected a barrage of calls as soon as I dialed the phones from the answering service. However, the phones were strangely silent. Everyone was obviously too busy calling relatives and friends, talking about the debris that had landed all over the county, including their own yards and pastures.

Anxious to learn more, I started making a few phone calls of my own. First I called the Sheriff's Department. Amy Marcantel confirmed what I already knew, that debris was falling everywhere.

I had already heard the rumors that an astronaut had been found, so I called my father to see what I needed to do if we did get called out. He wasn't home. This certainly didn't help my nerves. With ten years experience under my belt as a funeral director and embalmer, I felt I could handle just about anything that could be thrown my way. But a bona fide national disaster? I wasn't so sure. Now, I was suddenly convinced Dad had changed his mind and left for League City without bothering to call and leave instructions.

No sooner had my pacing begun than Dad walked through the back door. Silently thanking God he was here, I told him I could have handled it myself.

Although we weren't sure exactly what to prepare for, we did start making preparations. We called Doctor James Bruce, the pathologist in Lufkin, in an effort to secure a place equipped with a mortuary cooler. James was out of town for the weekend, so we tried the Jefferson County morgue; they said they would call us back.

We then began preparing our fleet. Despite being a relatively small rural funeral home, we have two black Cadillac hearses, a '91 and a '98, a black Ford Excursion for long distance transportation, and a white van as a flower vehicle. Due to our unusually close working relations with the Sabine County Sheriff's Department, both of our hearses and the Excursion are equipped with police radios. I loaded a pair of body bags, a box of gloves, and sheets into the '91 hearse, the van, and the Excursion. The hearse and the Excursion were each loaded with a cot, while the van was loaded with our 'jump cot'—a handy little collapsible stretcher, scarcely larger than a standard medical backboard.

While I prepared the vehicles, Dad made a trip to the sheriff's office. When he returned, he confirmed that a crewmember had been found.

Not long after he got back from the sheriff's office, Dad called in Debi Greene, an employee at the funeral home who was serving out her funeral director and embalmer's apprenticeship.

A few minutes after Debi arrived, our secretary Virginia White called and said she was on her way, and not long after that, Dad made another trip to the sheriff's office. When he returned, he told me everything that was said and assured me that he had offered our services, but I wasn't satisfied. As soon as his back was turned I hopped in my car and made my own trip up town.

At the Blan Greer Law Enforcement Center I found the beginning of the command organization. A small folding card table had been placed in the front lobby. A map of the county was lying across the table, with marks denoting the locations of known debris. Chief Deputy Chad Murray was in the lobby looking over the map. He directed me to Texas Department of Public Safety Sergeant Tommy Scales, who was coordinating the DPS officers, and therefore in charge of the sites until the federal government arrived. I was relieved; at that time my greatest fear was that an outsider would already have taken the reins and deemed our small rural funeral home too insignificant to take part in the recovery operation. But I had worked several accidents with Tommy, and he knew our funeral home was quite capable of handling any situation that came our way. I found Tommy outside the jail on his way over to the fire hall. I told him we had all our vehicles ready to go if he needed us. He said he would call us if it was up to him, but the FBI would be taking over the recovery of the crew as soon as they arrived; all state and local organizations were under strict orders not to touch anything.

He also made mention of the first outside misinterpretation of the local situation. An order had come in that the crew and all crew-related sites were to be guarded; the instructions were that the guards were to be state troopers only, not local officers. The problem was, there were only two DPS troopers in the entire county, Tommy Scales and Tim Saltzman, and they had their hands full trying to get everything organized. Luckily, Scales was successful in convincing them to allow him to use local resources. Hemphill Police Chief Roger McBride and Deputies Bob Cole and Brad Shirley were dispatched to Beckham Road.

The second site of the day—the crew-related site at Bob White's house, down Farm Road 2024—was another story; when it was reported to the officials at around noon, the press was already on the scene. However, during the extra time several DPS officers had come in from the outlying areas. Most of these troopers were being used to investigate reports of shuttle debris, but a couple of officers were dispatched to secure the scene at the White residence.

Seeing that I was of little help in Tommy's current situation, I returned to the funeral home. Time passed slowly that afternoon while we waited. When Dad received a call that afternoon we had become so used to meaningless and fruitless calls that no one really expected this one to be the call we had been waiting on. We continued the office chatter until he motioned for us to be quiet. The talking instantly ceased.

When the conversation was done, Dad hung up the phone, turned to me and said, "Let's go."

3
Bringing it Together

S ATURDAY WAS NORMALLY Greg Cohrs' day to sleep in; however, the long-time U.S. Forest Service employee's body inevitably rebelled at this deviation from his weekday routine, causing him to snore, toss, and turn in the last few hours of his sleep. In order to let his wife get some sleep, Greg usually moved into the spare bedroom on his fitful Saturday mornings.

He was in the extra bedroom when the loud boom and rumbling shook his house, bringing him, at least partially, out of his heavy slumber. His wife Sandra quickly made her way into the room and asked if he knew what the sound had been. Still half asleep, Greg replied that he thought it was the heater unit hitting a defrost cycle, but Sandra, being more awake, knew that this wasn't the case. For one thing, it had been a mild, cool night, but not cool enough for the central heat to cycle. Besides, there was simply no way their heater could have made such a racket.

While Greg tried to gather his thoughts, Sandra left the bedroom. She put on her housecoat and went out the back door to have a look outside. As Greg lay in bed listening to the continued booming and rumbling, his thoughts moved from the air conditioner to military tests at Fort Polk, some forty-five to sixty miles away. Then he began to think about 9/11 and suddenly became worried that what he heard might have been a nuclear explosion in Houston or New Orleans. He offered up a prayer that this wasn't the case.

When Sandra returned to the spare bedroom, she told Greg that when she stepped outside, she could hear strange crackling and popping noises in the air. Greg couldn't think of a single logical explanation for the sounds she was hearing.

Greg got out of bed and he and Sandra went into the living room and turned on the TV. As soon as they turned to the news channel it became apparent that what they had heard was the shattered remains of the Space Shuttle Columbia flying over the area. The Cohrs' hearts and prayers went out for the crewmembers and their families as they watched the developments on TV.

After watching the news for quite some time, Greg got up from the couch and started getting ready to do the daily chores. He realized the magnitude of the situation, but he had yet to realize that the crisis was such a local issue; he knew the shattered shuttle had gone overhead, but, at this time, he didn't know just how much of it had landed in the area. Greg knew the Forest Service would more than likely be activated for this crisis, even if it wasn't a local issue. Before leaving the house, Greg made a few phone calls. One of these calls was to Tom Zimmerman, the Fire Management Officer for the Sabine National Forest. Tom told Greg that he had already been contacted and was standing by awaiting instructions. From what he could tell, a considerable amount of debris had fallen in the area, and he was sure they would be called out today.

After he got off the phone, Greg put off his chores for a little while longer. He sat down at his computer and logged on to the Internet. He brought up the National Weather Service radars for Lake Charles, Shreveport, and Fort Polk. All of the radars showed a long cloudy red northwest-to-southeast line that stretched from Nacogdoches County from a point just west of Leesville, Louisiana. Hemphill was directly in the middle of the area shown by the radar images.

After searching the net for some time, trying to gain some insight into the situation, Greg finally returned to the TV. Soon he became restless and decided to get on with the daily chores. Just before noon, he called Tom Zimmerman and told him that he would be out, but he would have his cell phone. He made sure that Tom had his number, and then started out the door. Greg made it no farther than the back of his couch before his home phone rang.

It was Tracy White, calling from the local U. S. Forest Service District Ranger office. She said a USFS helicopter was en route from Lufkin to assist in locating fallen debris. Since he was familiar with the area, they wanted him on the chopper. With the chopper on its way, there was little time to spare. Without bothering to change into his uniform, Greg hurried out the door and headed up town to the Forest Service office.

* * *

As soon as Greg walked through the door, he heard the Forest Service's Lufkin dispatcher speaking to the chopper pilot over the radio. The dispatcher informed the pilot that Sabine County was now under Temporary Flight Restriction. The chopper would have to turn around and go back to Lufkin.

District Ranger Marcus Beard had another assignment in mind for Greg. He told him to go up to the Incident Command Post and establish a joint command with the Incident Commander.

Greg gathered up several Forest Service maps. He knew these would be useful, since they included much more detail on the maze of dirt roads and logging trails that crisscrossed the county. Before heading up to the command center, Greg made a quick trip to his house in order to change into his uniform.

* * *

Greg arrived at the ICP just after noon. The command structure had yet to be etched in stone and the activity at the fire hall was furious. While there was already a basic order to this chaos, to a newcomer it seemed like utter pandemonium. There were people in various state and local police uniforms mixed with the civilian volunteers in and around the open bays of the fire hall. Everyone was in a hurry, even if they weren't exactly sure what their duties were at the time.

Greg had been told to make contact with the Incident Commander, but at first it was difficult for him to find just who that was. He asked around and found out that Tom Maddox was one of the Co-Incident Commanders, but the sheriff was too busy to talk at the moment. Greg found Billy Ted Smith, the other Co-Incident Commander, and was told to contact Jamie Gunter, Billy Ted's right hand man in the Emergency Management Corps. Greg offered all the resources and personnel the Sabine National Forest had available.

Having worked several forest fires and natural disasters throughout his career, Greg was one of the few people in Sabine County who had not only been trained in Emergency Operations Procedures, but he also had experience in the field. Greg soon became the Branch Director for the ground search in the Sabine County Area. He and Jamie immediately got to work organizing the units that were responding to the various debris calls throughout the county. In a short time, they transformed these units into what would become the operation's Response Teams for the next two weeks. The newly organized teams included law enforcement and Forest Service officials. Much like the earlier responders, these teams were to be sent to the debris sites that were being called in. The Forest Service members would now take GPS readings of the debris so the items could be effectively recorded on a map that was kept at the Incident Command Post.

At first these groups didn't prove as efficient as Greg and Jamie had hoped. It was taking far too long for the units to secure and take the readings of one site, then move on to another location. As the groups came back to the ICP for more orders, Greg asked them what was taking so long. They replied that each time they made a response call, they were flagged down by people with information on additional sites. The teams would then stop at these sites and take all the necessary readings there as well. It was apparent to Greg and Jamie that these detours were the root of their problem. When the teams responded to these unauthorized calls, they were often responding to calls that were actually on someone else's list. This meant the teams were often responding to sites only to find that another team had already been there.

Another problem that the teams faced was the size of the area they were trying to cover. A team might be given an area to respond to in the Six Mile, and then have to run across the county to Bronson, which was about twenty miles away.

Greg and Jamie addressed these problems by telling the teams that they were only to respond to the sites that were assigned through the ICP. They also made a greater effort to see that the assignments were given out in clusters that were near the same general area. Like the rest of the operation, the Response Teams and the people dispatching them to sites had to learn as they went. There was no specific protocol for this type of accident. While many of the leaders had disaster training, nothing like this had ever happened.

* * *

While the Incident Management Team was certainly breaking new ground, there were instances when past experience played a key role. Almost five years ago to the day, Greg had served as Attack Incident Commander on the initial night that a peculiar natural disaster had struck East Texas, and as Operations Chief for many subsequent months. In the spring of 1998, a powerful straight wind blew a northwest to southeast swath, crossing the Sam Houston, Angelina, and Sabine National Forests. While the actual storm had lasted only fifteen to twenty minutes and no tornadoes had been spawned, the extremely high winds had caused serious damage. An estimated 250,000 to 400,000 trees had been blown down, with some areas having received damage similar to Hurricane Hugo in 1989. The fallen trees had blocked roads and severed power lines, affecting citizens throughout the entire region.

The Forest Service officials had gathered teams and sawed their way through the fallen trees from the Hemphill Ranger Station to their Dreka Workcenter, near Shelbyville. Once there, they had begun poring over the maps, trying to decide how to go about clearing all the roads and highways. They had picked out the areas that they thought were most in need—those areas completely isolated by fallen timber—and they had started to work. The plan was effective and the crews had been making progress, but by four in the morning, fatigue had begun taking its toll on the crews and everyone had just been beginning to realize the magnitude of the disaster: there was simply no way they could clear all the roads in one shift. It had been decided that the crews would go home and get some rest before returning to work. The next morning, the rested teams had picked up where they had left off, resuming a clearing operation that would eventually take months to complete.

It was with this in mind that Greg and Jamie decided to send the members of the response teams home for the night, even though they were making progress and there was a massive backlog of debris calls to address. There was a tremendous concern and desire to recover Columbia's crew, but it was obvious that the task was going to be enormous. He told them to go home and get some rest. They were to meet back at the ICP early the next morning. Although many law officers continued responding to calls on into the night, the ones who would be expected to work the day shift the next day went home. Sunday was going to be hectic enough without having to fight against sleep deprivation.

Greg and Jamie then sat down and began to work out a plan for Sunday's search.

First, they started making the map. Before Greg arrived, the operation had used a massive map of the county that had been created by printing several close-ups of the 911 maps from their computer and pasting them all together by hand. This map was approximately eight feet by eight feet, and had to be stretched out across several folding tables. This map showed both paved and dirt roads, creeks and the lake, as well as city and county boundaries, but the map did not have the detail of the Forest Service maps Greg had brought with him from the office. The Forest Service transportation system maps were used as a guide to locate the easiest travel routes to reported locations. Greg took GPS generated maps of Columbia-related materials and used them to plot some of the most critical sites of the day on the Sabine National Forest map. He noticed that the main path of debris seemed to run from the Chinquapin area of San Augustine County, through Bronson and through a point just south of Hemphill, near the Springhill area, with the crew-related sites near the center of the path. He focused on these critical finds and used them as the primary points on a two and a half to three mile wide path on either side of the northwest to southeast centerline, which ran through the center of the county. This was the primary area of concern. Next, Greg drew a much wider path, about six to seven miles on either side of the primary area; this was the secondary area of concern. By the time they were finished, they had greatly narrowed the initial search corridor to the area in which the remaining six crewmembers were likely to be found.

After the map was completed, the operation leaders sat down and began trying to plan out the next day's ground search. The problem with planning the search was that they knew the leadership personnel that would be available—Forest Service, Emergency Management Corps, Department of Public Safety, FBI, NASA, and other organizations—but they had no idea how many volunteers and searchers would turn up the following morning. They would have to do the balance of the planning in the morning, when they had a better knowledge of their resources.

At 11:30 p.m., Greg finally went home. He would have to be back at the ICP early the next morning to organize and supervise the first day's ground search.

4
Setting Protocol

S INCE WE KNEW we might be called out to both the crew site and the crew-related site, my father and I took two vehicles. He drove the Excursion and I followed in the '91 hearse. In hindsight, bringing the hearse might not have been such a good idea. For one thing, we would only be called on to work one site at a time, so only one vehicle was needed. Also, reporters were beginning to converge on the county in droves and the long black hearse stuck out like a sore thumb.

Instead of driving to the Law Enforcement Center, Dad continued to the new ICP, the fire hall. Currently all six bays were empty and the doors were wide open.

Several officials from the city of Hemphill had been instrumental in the initial creation of the Command Post at the Hemphill fire hall, including Mayor Robert Hamilton, City Manager Don Iles, and Fire Chief D. B. Chance. The fire trucks were moved across the street in order to clear out the bays, and tables and chairs were moved in and set up. At first one of the bays was roped off for the media, which was beginning to trickle in and would soon swamp the area. It was quickly decided that this was too close for comfort and the media center was moved across the street.

The first problem in setting up the Incident Command Post was communications. There was only one phone line in the entire fire hall, and it was apparent that several more would be needed. The local phone company was contacted and about a dozen new phone lines were installed by nightfall. This helped ease the situation, but insufficient communication would remain a problem throughout the entire operation.

By noon, Billy Ted Smith arrived from Beaumont. One of his first actions was to ask Sabine County Judge Jack Leath to declare a state of emergency. This gave the local law enforcement agency greater control over the situation and allowed them to request aid from the state and federal level.

At that point the command structure began to take shape, with Billy Smith and Tom Maddox serving as Co-Incident Commanders, and Jamie Gunter as the Operations Chief. Hemphill and Newton Counties had only been part of the Emergency Management Corps since December, so very few Sabine County residents were trained in mass emergency operations. As a result, many of the initial positions were filled by Jasper County law enforcement officials, with Sabine County officials serving as liaisons for the various local departments. The main exception was the local U.S. and Texas Forest Service Personnel. Several of these state and federal employees had not only received emergency management training, but had experience in using the command structure while fighting forest fires and other natural disasters.

Not long after the ICP had been established, Terry Lane, an FBI agent out of Lufkin, arrived in Hemphill. Not long after Terry's appearance at the Command Post, a second FBI agent arrived on the scene—Shane Ball. Once the command structure was firmly established, Shane would coordinate the FBI's operations at the Command Post, while Terry coordinated the field operations. They would become an invaluable asset to the most important aspect of the operation—the recovery of Columbia's crew.

Although the official federal state of emergency had been declared much earlier in the morning, it was around noon before the fax reached Sabine County. Emergency assistance under Title V of the Stafford Act would be provided, as it was deemed necessary by the Federal Emergency Management Agency—FEMA. This assistance was to be provided at one-hundred percent federal funding. The declaration listed thirty-eight Texas Counties and several Louisiana Parishes, but the primary focus of the operation would be on five East Texas Counties—Anderson, Rusk, Nacogdoches, San Augustine, and Sabine.

* * *

Dad parked across the street from the fire hall, and I pulled up in front of the first bay door. We located Tommy Scales, who directed us to a man in an FBI shirt, Terry Lane. Dad, Terry, Tommy, Chad Murray, and Sheriff Tom Maddox talked over the situation while I looked on in silence. They agreed that the crew-related sites needed to be cleared as soon as possible—the media had already discovered the site at Bob White's, and it was only a matter of time before word got out about the site down Beckham Road. However, NASA had yet to arrive, and they had specifically requested that these sensitive sites were to remain undisturbed until a NASA official was present.

Moving from the funeral home to the command center had only changed our surroundings. While the deputies and DPS troopers continued making mad dashes back and forth across the county investigating debris sites, my father and I continued waiting to be called into action. During this lull I spoke to several longtime neighbors and friends and realized during these conversations that just about everyone, from the volunteers bringing food to the people running the operation, was still in shock over what had happened and what *was* happening. The shuttle disaster itself was difficult to believe, but the fact that this drama was playing itself out in our sleepy little town was just unbelievable.

After we had been at the ICP for an hour, the sound of a helicopter broke the monotony. I stepped outside the building and saw a low-flying chopper slowly circling the command post as if it was looking for a place to land. I overheard someone saying the helicopter was from NASA and that a pair of astronauts was onboard. Since the helicopter couldn't land here, it was rerouted to the football field, across town.

* * *

Sabine County Reserve Deputy Jamie Williams had been called in that morning to help with the crisis. After spending the morning responding to debris calls, he had taken a break to go to the high school gym to watch two of his nieces play in a "Little Dribblers" basketball game. Jamie had just sat down in the bleachers and taken his first bite of a barbecue sandwich, his first meal of the day, when Robert "Pudding" Wright, one of the sponsors of the local Little Dribblers, entered the gym and began scanning the stands. Jamie figured they were looking for him, so he began wolfing down his sandwich as fast as he could, hoping he could finish before they spotted him. The hard-to-miss uniform gave him away before he was halfway through; Pudding saw Jamie and motioned for him. Still trying to swallow a little over half a barbecue sandwich, Jamie made his way down to the floor.

"We need you to take the astronauts up to the Command Post," Pudding said as Jamie approached.

"What astronauts?"

"The two who just landed on the football field."

Jamie had heard the helicopter, but he had assumed it was part of the search.

Pudding continued, "We figured it would look better if you took them, since you're in uniform."

"I'm not in a patrol car. I'm in my pickup."

"That's fine."

Jamie shrugged, "Okay then, where are they?"

"Here they come," Pudding nodded toward the area behind Jamie.

When Jamie turned around there were two men in blue NASA jumpsuits approaching from behind him. After everyone had been introduced, the group started out the door toward Jamie's pickup.

When the astronauts arrived at the ICP that afternoon, many people imagined that NASA would take over the operation; however, these astronauts were not present as the vanguard of a federal takeover. They had voluntarily shouldered the heavy task of recovering the remains of their friends and coworkers. They were here to see that the crewmembers were handled with the dignity that they deserved.

Despite the grimness of their mission, these astronauts still managed an air of respect and kindness toward the local volunteers. Not only did these two men set the tone of professionalism and reverence that would prevail throughout the operation, but they also unconsciously began the development of a strong tie between the locals and NASA.

* * *

Once they arrived at the ICP the astronauts met with Terry, Sheriff Maddox and my father outside the fire hall before continuing into the meeting hall. Once again I played the part of the silent onlooker. This was the first time I heard mention of a piece of unofficial protocol that would remain true throughout the operation. From now on, as soon as a crewmember or a crew-related site was found, an astronaut would be sent to the location. This astronaut would stay at the site as an honor guard throughout the recovery and even during transportation. When this discussion was finished, Terry Lane and Astronaut Marc Kelly drove out to Beckham Road while the second astronaut departed for San Augustine County.

After the astronauts left the fire hall, I began to feel the return of that sinking feeling that we would be left out. When they left, Terry had seemed in favor of at least using us for transportation, but Marc seemed hesitant. However, they weren't gone long before the call came in for us to come out to the site at Beckham Road.

Right before we left, Jason Pearson, an employee at the funeral home who had been helping out with the Six Mile

Volunteer Fire Department, pulled up to the command post. He followed us in his pickup. We took a slightly longer route out of town and down Springhill Road in order to throw off any media that might be watching.

* * *

Police ribbon was stretched across the road, blocking traffic just around a curve so a person who drove up wouldn't be able to see the site without crossing the police line. As a result, we couldn't see the site until we were out of our cars and around the corner. An ambulance and several patrol cars, some county, some Hemphill Police, and a few newly arrived DPS cars, were parked across the site on the other side of the second line of yellow tape. A yellow rain slicker lay stretched out near the center of the blue rock road.

Dad discussed the situation with Terry and Marc, while Jason and I spoke with Paramedic David Whitmire and Hemphill Police Chief Roger McBride. Once we had been brought up to speed, Terry and Marc resumed taking down information about the site.

While we were waiting, something happened that served as a clear indication just how out of sorts I was on that first day. While jotting down his notes, Terry asked which way was east. I promptly located the sun and pointed at it. Dad shook his head and pointed vaguely in the opposite direction. "No, it's that way."

"The sun rises in the west," I replied. Then I wasn't so sure. "Doesn't it?"

"No, it rises in the east," Terry commented without looking up from his notes.

I suddenly wished I could find a hole to hide in.

After they thoroughly documented the site, Marc and Terry decided to go ahead and transport the crewmember. Although we lacked refrigeration facilities, Dad offered the use of our embalming room for temporary storage. Terry said this wouldn't be necessary. The FBI had already been in contact with Dr. Bruce, who had okayed the use of his facilities.

I went to the hearse to get the jump cot, a body bag, and a box of gloves. Right after I had returned to the site and began to make preparations for the removal, Marc spoke up. He asked if we could have a minister or a chaplain come out and say a few words. Dad suggested Fred Raney, pastor of the First Baptist Church of Hemphill. Roger McBride called the ICP, and, as it turned out, Fred was there.

During the brief wait for Fred's arrival, an orange Coast Guard helicopter began slowly circling the site, staying just over the treetops at a distance where the breeze from its whirling blades' rotor wash was barely felt on our faces. As I looked up at the slow-moving chopper, I began to realize the grim reality of this situation. Glancing around at my companions, I saw several other faces staring up at the helicopter with a look of wonder about them. At that point, I believe the realization of this tragedy was beginning to sink in on all of us.

When Fred arrived, we made a circle around the raincoat-covered crewmember and lowered our heads. Marc, Terry, Jason, Roger, Fred, David, my father and I were present for this, the first of many prayers that would be said over the bodies of our fallen heroes. Marc's suggestion that a prayer be said over the crewmembers became another part of the respect that was shown throughout the operation. Brother Fred Raney would become an important part of the recovery; he would be called out to every site to give a prayer. Even the crew-related finds were to be given the same respect as the crewmembers themselves. Also, his prayers were taken from the Old Testament out respect to the crew's diverse religious background. After the prayer, Dad and I carefully placed the crewmember into the body bag.

After the crewmember was secured on the jump cot, Terry, Marc, and Dad turned their attention to the second site. They decided to leave the body inside the car while they made the second recovery. In order to keep an astronaut with the remains at all time, Marc would accompany Dad in the hearse.

My father and I then lifted the jump cot from the ground and started toward the hearse. The load wasn't heavy, but, out of respect for a fallen friend, Marc insisted on helping my father and me place the cot in the hearse. Once the cot was loaded, Dad told Jason to take me back to the command post to get the Excursion then return and assist in the search of the surrounding area.

Jason and I made a flying trip back to the ICP. When we got there, Jason had to leave us once again so he could help with the fire department, so I made the return trip alone. On my way back down Springhill Road, I met the hearse on its way back to the command center.

* * *

Back at the first site, DPS officers and a handful of volunteers were wading into the brush around the site. I spoke briefly with Roger before wandering off by myself in an effort to clear my cluttered head. I soon realized that there wasn't much more I could do at this site, so I asked Roger to radio in and see if I could return to the ICP. Five minutes later I was on my way back into Hemphill.

* * *

When I returned to the Incident Command Post I found the hearse had been pulled inside the yellow ribbon. There were more cameras than before, and the presence of the hearse had stirred the media considerably.

I parked across the street from the command post. Much to my surprise, I wasn't able to dart across the road. Heavy traffic in downtown Hemphill was unheard of, but there I was, waiting for someone to stop and let me cross. I recognized most of the faces behind the wheels; the majority of the vehicles were driven by the curious and concerned locals who had come out to see what was going on. However, there were already a number of unfamiliar faces and an ever-increasing number of DPS patrol cars.

After I made it across the street to the ICP, Dad told me there was another crew-related find in San Augustine County. They were trying to coordinate it so they could make the recovery down Farm Road 2024, then roll from there straight to San Augustine, and then continue to Dr Bruce's in Lufkin.

Dad told me to stay with the hearse and then went inside the fire hall's meeting room. After discussing the final preparations with Shane Ball, Dad returned and climbed into the hearse. Seeing this, one of the volunteers thought he was ready to leave and lowered the yellow ribbon. However, Dad was still waiting on Marc, who was finishing some business inside the fire hall. As soon as the yellow ribbon came down the press surged forward with cameras and microphones, barraging my father with questions concerning the recovery of the astronaut. Most of the officers who had been present earlier had been dispatched about the county to debris sites, leaving the ICP manned mostly by the various volunteer fire departments. While Dad answered the only way possible—"No comment"—I started toward the meeting room to try and find someone with the authority to get the press on the other side of the perimeter. I located Chad Murray inside the building, near the map. He returned with me to the hearse and he was able to get the reporters away from the vehicle.

In hindsight, this wasn't exactly the crisis it seemed at the time. There were probably no more than a dozen reporters, but my nerves were still borderline-panicky; to me, it seemed like a breach in a siege.

Not long after the yellow tape barrier had been restored, Marc came from the meeting room and joined Dad in the hearse. An escort was arranged and they were off to the second scene, leaving me behind at the ICP.

* * *

When the hearse arrived at Bob White's, the media were there in full force. Still, the site was secured and the best they could manage was to take pictures from a distance. As before, Fred said a brief prayer, and the crew-related item was photographed before Dad respectfully placed it in its own body bag. The media filmed away as Dad and Reverend Raney loaded the body bag into the back of the hearse. In fact, a clip from this scene played repeatedly on CNN over the next couple of days.

This would be the last time the media would make it out to one of our sites.

* * *

Back at the ICP I found myself once again anxious to find something to do. Volunteers were arriving with food, so I helped set up the tables. One of the volunteers offered me a sandwich, but, despite the fact I hadn't eaten all day, I wasn't hungry.

Dad had told me to stay close in case they found another crewmember. In truth, he probably meant for me to go home and wait by the phone, but I still wanted to be close to the action. I milled around the ICP for the remainder of the day, but when darkness came I finally decided it was time to leave. I touched base with Shane, gave him my work and home phone numbers, and then returned to the funeral home.

When we closed the office, I forwarded the funeral home phones to my house instead of to the answering service. If they called for me, I wanted to be able to respond with as little delay as possible.

5

Into the Woods

WHILE GREG COHRS and Jamie Gunter organized and mapped out the search effort for Sunday, preparations were already underway to convert the local VFW Post into the operation's Volunteer Staging Area. Roger Gay, the current Veterans of Foreign Wars Post Commander, and his wife Belinda organized the VFW hall's kitchen for the coming task of feeding the masses of volunteers and government workers who would be arriving throughout the operation. The kitchen at the VFW post was ideal for the task. It was designed to prepare meals not only for the regular meetings and weekly bingo games, but also for various banquets and other major functions that happened throughout the year. All of the equipment was heavy duty and in great shape. Rows of tables and folding chairs were available in the main hall. Roger and Belinda were perfect for the task of organizing just such an operation, and not just because Roger happened to be the Post Commander. Roger and Belinda were also the owners of "Fat Fred's," a gas station and restaurant combination in Hemphill, and, more importantly, Belinda ran a catering service that operated out of the restaurant.

On the day the shuttle went down, the makeshift kitchen crew had worked diligently to feed the volunteers who came and went throughout the day. However, Sunday morning would be their first meal that would have to be prepared and served at a set time. This would be the real test.

* * *

On Sunday morning the kitchen was organized into an assembly line. The eggs were broken and placed in a blender for a quick scrambling. They were then poured onto the kitchen's large griddle. All in all, sixty dozen eggs were prepared on that first morning, and this would be the lightest day. At the operation's height the cooks would be preparing 300 dozen eggs a morning.

As the volunteer searchers arrived they passed through a buffet where they were offered a full breakfast. Eggs, grits, sausage, and toast were brought out as it came out of the kitchen. Coffee and juice were offered at the end of the buffets, as were various jars of jelly. An assortment of pastry items that had been donated by people in the community also graced the table. It was impressive that so much organized work could come out of the chaos and confusion of the day before.

* * *

Cars and pickups began turning into the VFW hall, now know as the Volunteer Staging Area, well before sunrise Sunday morning. By six o'clock, the parking lot was full and cars were beginning to fill the nearby rodeo arena parking lot.

Bob Morgan wasn't sure where the call for volunteers had originated. On the night before, the request for volunteers to meet at the VFW hall at six o'clock in the morning had passed by word of mouth to all the volunteer firefighters who were still at the ICP. Bob was the chief of the Six Mile Volunteer Fire Department, so it was his duty to see that all the firefighters from Six Mile knew that they were going to be called out to search the woods the next morning. When he returned home, he got on the phone and called the members who had not been present at the Command Center.

Bob had been sick over the past week and he was still warding off the lingering effects of a flu-bug that had been going around the county. However, he felt honored to be able to take part in this operation; there was no way he was going to stay home in bed. Around the world, millions of eyes were turned to East Texas, and many hearts were pouring out prayers and best wishes. While the vast majority of America looked on with heavy hearts, we were the lucky few who were able to get our hands dirty for the cause.

Bob Morgan had moved to Six Mile, a small community in Sabine County, after retiring from the Internal Revenue Service. In the late eighties, not long after he moved to the area, Bob had been instrumental in founding the Six Mile Volunteer Fire Department. Throughout the years, the fire department grew from a single old tanker truck loaned from the Texas Forest Service and stored in a member's garage to a very active organization boasting three trucks and twenty active members.

As the Six Mile volunteers arrived, they gathered at one of the hall's long tables. Aside from the occasional question about the search operation, the usually lively group ate their breakfast in silence. A sense of shock still prevailed over the entire county. As Saturday had played itself out, some of the shock had slipped away, but the next morning it was back. It was almost as if they had expected to wake up and find out it had all been a dream. However, the feeling on this Sunday morning was different than it had been the day before; the volunteers realized that yesterday's frantic mood had matured into a hard determination to help in every way possible. It was time to get to work.

* * *

When Greg arrived Sunday morning with the maps and plans, he was pleasantly surprised with the turnout. Even with such short notice, around two-hundred volunteers had shown up. The Forest Service officials came from the Sabine, Angelina, and Davy Crocket Ranger Districts. The other searchers were members of the local volunteer fire departments, employees of the Sabine River Authority, the FBI, DPS, and the Texas Forest Service. There were also several volunteers present who weren't affiliated with any group whatsoever; they had simply discovered there was a need and had come on their own accord.

The first order of the day was a morning prayer, given by Brother Fred Raney. Everyone paused from their breakfast and lowered their heads while Fred blessed the food and asked for guidance in the day's search.

After everyone had eaten, the ladies in the kitchen began clearing the tables while the searchers were given tags to identify themselves as members of the operation. These first tags were nothing more than black writing on white laminated cards reading, *Shuttle Incident Search Team Member, February 2, 2003*.

While the cards were being passed out, Greg met with the U.S. and Texas Forest Service personnel and other group leaders in order to work out the details of the plan. Greg divided the Sabine Ranger District personnel into four groups and supplemented these groups with members of the other ranger districts. Also, the teams were divided so that each group included members with superior forestry skills. Four Forest Service personnel were picked according to their superior leadership, forestry, and navigational skills and were placed in command of each group: Jamie Sowell, Group 1; Tom Zimmerman, Group 2; Shane Neal, Group 3; and Bobi Stiles, Group 4. Michael Bradberry of the Texas Department of Transportation served as the direct supervisor of Groups 1 and 2 while Jasper Police Officer Mike Poindexter supervised Groups 3 and 4.

The plan was to drop Bradberry's groups off at Beckham Road, near the first crew member site, while Poindexter's groups were to start near the crew-related site on Farm Road 2024. From their starting points, both groups would proceed in a northwestern direction on either side of the centerline. The volunteers were then to walk in an orderly line through incredibly dense terrain, keeping a constant eye toward the ground for any pieces of shuttle debris. If a searcher located a piece of debris, he was to call out for one of the U.S. Forest Service officers following behind the line. The line would stop while the debris was marked with ribbon, the GPS coordinates taken, and a description listed before the line moved on. If a searcher stumbled onto one of the crewmembers or any crew-related debris, the same procedure was to be followed, except that a volunteer would be left behind until an FBI agent or a NASA official arrived to relieve them. A Forest Service member was also stationed at each end of the lines, flagging the outer boundaries in order to mark the area that had been searched.

In order to get so many people out to the starting point, several buses had been brought into the county during the night. Some of these buses were supplied by the state and some were on loan from local school districts. Later in the week a few chartered buses would be arriving.

Even though the transportation was available, the volunteers weren't immediately put to work. While the volunteer groups were being organized at the VFW hall, employees of the U.S. Forest Service and the Texas Parks and Wildlife were still going over the final details of the search. The volunteers were unaware that the Forest Service was busily planning their route; as the minutes ticked by, many of the volunteers began grumbling at the delay, but no one went home.

* * *

Bradley Byley would be leaving early the next morning for a job and wouldn't be back in town for weeks. However, he wanted to do all he could to help in the short time he had left. He arrived at the VFW hall just as the volunteers were beginning to load into the buses. He located Michael Bradberry and offered to get a group of five to ten people on horseback together to help with the search. Michael said they could use all the help they could get and asked Bradley to meet them down Beckham Road at 9:30 a.m.

As Bradley started back out the door to his truck, he glanced at his watch. It was already 9:15. With such short notice, there was no way he would be able to get a decent sized group together. He was going to be hard-pressed just to hook up his own trailer and get his own horse loaded.

On the way home, Bradley had just enough time to use his cell phone to contact one other rider—Dale Wilkerson. Dale said he would meet Bradley down Beckham Road.

Fifteen minutes just wasn't enough time to load and saddle his horse, and then drive out to Beckham Road. Bradley was on his way to the drop off point about thirty minutes later, worrying that he might be left behind. However, when he got to the starting area, he found that the search had not begun. He and Dale unloaded their horses near the end of the blacktop and rode on down to where the searchers were gathering.

There was still some time before the search teams were stretched into a long line and led into the woods, so the two men sat atop their horses and waited. As Bradley watched the line slowly take form, he became impressed by the people present for the search—not just the number of people, but by the *type* of people who were present. Most of the volunteers were affiliated with one of the local volunteer fire departments, but many were individuals who had simply arrived at the staging area that morning to lend a hand. Some people didn't even know about the search until that morning; these had stopped whatever they were doing and traveled out to meet the search group at the end Beckham Road. Bankers and lawyers were lined up to search the woods beside loggers and farmers. Men and women, old and young, all races—everybody there was grouped into one classification: "volunteer."

* * *

On Saturday, the day before, the local high schools had been contacted to provide transportation for the volunteers. Sheriff Tom Maddox had at one time been a member of the school board for the West Sabine Independent School District in Pineland, so he was well acquainted with the three men on their maintenance crew. Before noon, before the Incident Command Post was even fully functional at the fire hall, Tom contacted Joe Simmons and asked if West Sabine could supply a few buses for the search operation the next morning.

Joe then contacted West Sabine's interim superintendent, Charlie Wilson, and asked permission to use three of the buses for the recovery operation. Charlie gave Joe permission to do whatever he thought was necessary. Joe then contacted the other two members of the maintenance crew, Charlie Creech and Murray Kilgore, and asked if they would like to drive for the volunteers. All three men were currently suffering from the same flu-bug that was ailing Bob and much of the rest of the county, but they volunteered nonetheless.

Early Sunday morning, Joe, Charlie, and Murray had met at the bus barn. At six o'clock they left for Hemphill, arriving in time to eat breakfast with the rest of the volunteers.

It was after nine o'clock when the volunteers were loaded onto the buses provided by Hemphill and West Sabine schools, and it was almost ten before the volunteers were taken to Beckham Road. Once the searchers were unloaded, the buses were taken to where Beckham Road turns into Springhill Road. The drivers parked along the side of the road and waited throughout the day for word to come to pick up the volunteers.

* * *

After thirty minutes of organizing the line, the volunteers finally began pushing slowly and steadily into the woods. These volunteers knew that they had a difficult job ahead of them, but they weren't fully aware of the challenges they would face until they actually set foot in the woods. To understand the obstacles they had to overcome, one has to understand the terrain in which they were searching. For one thing, the East Texas piney woods defy the laws of geometry in that the shortest distance from one point to another is very seldom a straight line. A person walking through these woods can come upon several obstacles, such as bogs, marshes, thickets, and creeks, not to mention the occasional wild boar. Under normal circumstances, these obstacles would be avoided by taking a longer, yet much easier, path around them.

However, the men and women of the search groups didn't have that luxury. They had to beat a straight and steady path through whatever terrain was ahead. Creeks that meandered back on themselves had to be crossed as many times as they crossed a searcher's path; several of the searchers returned that afternoon soaked from the chest down from having to cross a creek in a deep area. Machetes, pocket knives, and whatever else was available were used to hack through the densest of underbrush. And throughout the first two weeks of the operation, there were several run-ins with the local wildlife; fortunately, none of these encounters resulted in injury.

One such run-in happened early that first morning while Bob was working his way through some of the heavy underbrush. The members of Bobi Stiles' Group 4 were walking with about ten feet between each searcher. Before they entered the thicket, Bob could see down the line some distance, but once he was in the thicket he could barely see the searcher on either side of him. As he pressed forward into the brush, Bob heard movement ahead of him. Without giving him more than a few seconds to react, a large doe burst through the brush and started his way with a young spotted fawn trailing along behind her. The deer charged to within ten feet of him before it suddenly stopped; it glanced around, as if confused, and then retreated into the brush. Bob continued only a few feet farther before he found the deer's abandoned bed of twigs and underbrush.

A second, much milder encounter happened when a Six Mile volunteer pointed out a water moccasin sunning on a rock beside the creek. In the country, most of us have the notion that the discovery of a poisonous snake near one's home means your pets, livestock, and/or children could be in danger. The reaction of most of the group was a common reaction for the area—they started looking for a stick or rock they could use to kill the snake. Bobi told them to leave it alone; she said it wasn't hurting anyone. This didn't exactly set well with Jason Pearson, who has a mild phobia of snakes and firmly believes they should all be put to death on sight. But Bobi insisted, and the volunteers listened to their group leader. The snake was left to sun in peace while the humans trudged on through the woods.

* * *

Unlike the searchers on foot, the two mounted searchers weren't put on the line. The officials in charge of the search were afraid that the riders might miss something from their high vantage point. It soon became apparent that Bradley and Dale were very useful in another unforeseen area—communication. Not only were radios in short supply on the line, the reception in the woods was poor at best. Cell phones were all but useless; reception ranged from terrible to nothing at all. Considering the fact that when an item was found, the entire line was supposed to stop while GPS coordinates were taken, communication was very important. Often simply passing the word down the line would suffice, but the thick underbrush often made such communication slow and unreliable. Also, there were times that one group leader simply needed to speak with another leader. It was soon discovered that Bradley and Dale served as perfect messengers. They stayed busy throughout the day trotting from one end of the line to the other, delivering messages to and from the group leaders.

Also, when the line entered a particularly thick area, the riders were able to ride along the back of the line, using their higher vantage point to see into the thick brush where the searchers might have missed.

At one point, Bradley's horse also had to serve as a makeshift ambulance. One of the women on the line overexerted herself and was overcome with fatigue. Bradley placed her in the saddle and walked her back to Beckham Road, where an ambulance was waiting.

* * *

In the early afternoon, the searchers halted for a break. Red

Cross volunteers worked their way through the brush to bring the weary searchers their lunch, in the form of sandwich bags that had been prepared back at the VFW hall as well as military EMRE rations. Jason tried one of the EMRE kits and wasn't impressed in the least. In fact, he commented to one of the other searchers that he firmly believed the government fed these kits to the soldiers just to make them mad, hoping it would make them fight harder.

While they were taking their break, the traffic on Bob's handheld radio increased as the preparations for the first crew-related recovery of the day got underway on the other side of the county. Through the static, Bob was able to make out that the newly arrived FBI recovery team was requesting four-wheelers. He knew Jason and Todd had arrived this morning with their four-wheelers in the back of their pickups. Bob hadn't seen Todd since the beginning of the break, but Jason was nearby. He asked Jason if he would be interested in helping out. Jason replied that he would and he was sure Todd would help as well. The only problem would be locating a ride back to the staging area, where they left their pickups.

Bob got on the radio and informed the ICP that he had two volunteers with four-wheelers and he would send them out as soon as he could find a way to get them out of the woods. As it turned out, they were lucky the call happened during the break. At any other time it would have been almost impossible to get them out. As it was, Jason located Todd at the Red Cross wagon, stuffing his pockets with water and fruit. They were then able to thumb a ride back to the VFW hall with the Red Cross crew.

After their short break, the searchers hit the woods once more. They were only halfway through with the first day of searching. There was still a lot of work ahead.

* * *

The search continued until late that afternoon. Just before nightfall, the buses were sent out to pick up the volunteers and take them back to the staging area. A full supper was waiting for them when they returned. After they had eaten, most of the volunteers wearily made their way home for some much needed rest.

Once everybody was out of the woods, the fire chiefs and group leaders met with the command personnel to discuss the day's activities. Questions were raised concerning the length of the line—if they were spread out ten feet apart, how much were they missing? It was suggested that the lines separate into smaller teams, with a team leader over each section; that way communication with the search coordinators wouldn't be so difficult. Judging by the sheer amount of debris found, the first day's search could be considered a success, but these volunteers weren't going to sit on their laurels and say good was good enough. There was room for improvement, so the group leaders and the volunteers spoke up. Even more importantly, the coordinators listened.

* * *

All in all, the operation had matured considerably over the last twenty-four hours. While the searchers were in the woods, the incident leaders were tending to operational decisions as they arose, as well as mapping the area and working out plans for the next day. With all the new agencies and officials coming and going, there was still some evidence of friction of command in the peripheral portions of the operation. Incident Management training indicates that an operation should develop from the top down and the ground up; that is, the command structure grows as the need arises. This was readily apparent on the second day as the inner core of the operation's leaders, their liaisons, and the teams in the fields were already beginning to develop efficiency, while several of the outer branches of the growing command structure and newly arrived organizations were having difficulties establishing themselves. In short, this was a local operation that was quickly growing into the focal point of what would become the largest ground search in the history of the United States—so of course there were going to be growing pains.

The coordinators were building the command structure on these first two days. They would later recall that these were hectic, confusing days. Ironically, many of the local individuals serving as liaisons and assistants at the Incident Command Post would consider this second day the most organized in the entire operation. The obvious reason is that the necessary rapid growth of the operation kept the leaders of the operation on their feet that day, but the smaller command structure was simply more readily accessible.

Another reason that the initial command structure was so efficient in the eyes of the locals was that they were working with people they knew. The Incident Commanders and their staff, all of the leaders in the Operations and Logistic Sections, and most of the liaisons were from Sabine or Jasper County. Tom Maddox, Billy Ted Smith, and Stanley Christopher made up the upper Incident Command, while Greg Cohrs, Jamie Gunter, Michael Bradberry, Mike Poindexter, Buddy Rector, Don Eddings, and Mark Allen—all residents of Sabine or Jasper County—were over the most crucial portions of the command structure. Locals also served in other positions in the Incident Command Post. Sabine County Judge Jack Leath was a constant presence at the command center. City Manager Don Iles was also at the fire hall from daylight until well after dark, his simple official title as liaison for the City of Hemphill not doing justice to the effort he put forth. Hemphill Police Chief Roger McBride served as a liaison for the Hemphill Police Department; he also was responsible for cataloging and storing the items that were brought in by locals who did not realize they weren't supposed to touch the debris. Jasper County Sheriff Billy Rowles, who was present in liaison and advisory roles in the beginning, would later become the Branch Director of the water search. Over the first three days of the search, it had evolved into a complex but very efficient operation. These local officials played a large part in the organization that made the operation run so smoothly.

Concern for public safety was still a top priority, but the frantic rumor-fueled fear of the first day was gone. In its place was caution based on facts. Near mid-afternoon, the DPS headquarters in Austin sent a fax to all law enforcement branches stating that all public and private school administrators in the path of the shuttle were to be contacted to determine if there was debris on the roofs or grounds of any of the schools. As a precautionary measure, if debris was present, the school was to be closed until the debris could be removed.

Rumors continued to float around that the Department of Defense would be taking over. This greatly concerned many of the local coordinators. The command structure that had been set up using local manpower and FEMA guidelines was working remarkably well, and they saw no need for a change. Monday would see the arrival of the first units of the National Guard. This new manpower was greatly appreciated, but some felt that this would be the first step in the DOD's takeover of the operation. Only time would tell what the next day would bring.

* * *

That night, when Bob finally got home and took the load off his feet, he found that his legs were killing him. He was in great shape for a man of seventy years, but this kind of heavy walking was taking its toll. The next morning quite a few volunteers wouldn't show up, many of them much younger and in much better physical condition than Bob, but Bob would be back at the VFW hall at six in the morning, ready to go. In fact, four of the Six Mile volunteer firefighters were over sixty-five years old. All four of them returned to the line the next day.

6

With Dignity and Respect

O N THE SAME morning that the volunteers were preparing for their first day in the field, we were once again shorthanded at the funeral home. Our secretary, Virginia White, came in to keep the office, but our apprentice embalmer, Debi Greene, was out of town and Jason was volunteering in the woods. At any moment we could be called out, but we couldn't just put a halt to our business and pick it up when the crisis passed. We decided that if we received a call to help with the operation we would both respond until our duties took us outside the county. At that point we decided that Dad would go and I would remain behind to answer calls for the funeral home.

Around noon we decided to switch around the supplies in the vehicles. The first day of the operation had proved that we needed to use the vehicles that were equipped with police radios. We weren't actually talking on the radios so much as simply using them as scanners, monitoring the communication back and forth from the sites to the command center. The supplies were taken out of the van, and I transferred the two body bags and the jump cot to the Excursion.

I mentioned to my father that we only had four body bags remaining, but before we could contact our embalming supply company, the handheld radio on his desk came to life. We had been listening for most of the morning while the officers were dispatched to the debris sites, but this was different. We could tell they were excited about something. They certainly didn't come out and say they had found another crewmember, but there was no doubt that they had found something very significant. Several units, including a newly arrived FBI recovery team, were dispatched south of town, to Fire Tower Road, halfway between Hemphill and Six Mile.

The call wasn't long in coming. We were told to report to the command center for instructions.

* * *

We knew from Saturday's experience that the hearse drew too much attention from the media. We climbed into the Excursion and left the hearse at the funeral home. On the way to the command center I found that I wasn't half as nervous as I had been the day before. While the seriousness of the situation was still foremost in my mind, the overall shock had begun to wear off.

I noticed the changes to the Incident Command Post before I even got out of the Excursion. A trooper was standing guard at the fire hall's entrance—the ICP was now restricted from unauthorized entry. Two buses, several vans, and command vehicles for various departments and organizations were now parked in front of the building, and the metal bay doors had been closed. DPS troopers and other men in various uniforms stood outside the building. The tall, windowless headquarters looked like a fort.

Inside, I found more changes. The place was still just as crowded, but the crowd itself had changed considerably. Most of the volunteers were now out at the VFW Post, which was now the Volunteer Staging Area. In fact, my Dad and I were just about the only people in the building not wearing some sort of uniform.

When we located Shane Ball he asked if we were familiar with Fire Tower Road. We were. It's an old dirt road running off of Highway 87 about five miles south of Hemphill. He told us to go to the beginning of the road, and a car would meet us at the highway to lead us in.

* * *

The county patrol car ahead of us continued straight down the Fire Tower Road for about a mile before turning right down another dirt road. We didn't continue all the way to the Yellowpine fire tower; our escort turned onto a dirt road to the left about halfway down to the Fire Tower. We followed the car until the woods opened up to a large clearing.

That morning Charlie and Tammy Waldrop, the owners of one of the three houses in the clearing, had gone into the woods on their four-wheeler to look for debris. They discovered a crewmember on the farthest edge of their land, which bordered the Sabine National Forest. They immediately returned home and called the sheriff's department.

As soon as they arrived, Terry Lane, Marc Kelley, and two Texas Game Wardens asked Charlie to lead them to the site. As usual, Marc remained with the crewmember from that point on. Terry and the two game wardens stayed with him. Charlie and Tammy returned to their house while Terry made a cell phone call to get an FBI recovery team en route to the scene. Then he made another call to the command center, telling the dispatcher to contact us.

When we pulled up, the FBI team was already there. We parked the Excursion and got out. I recognized Chad Murray, Fred Raney, and Tommy Scales. Also present was a man wearing a sidearm and a uniform I'd never seen before; the patch on his shoulder identified him as a NASA security officer.

An attractive lady with a long ponytail introduced herself as Debbie, the head of the FBI recovery team. My father and I joined in the ongoing discussion concerning how to get the recovery team's equipment to the scene and how to recover the crewmember once we got there.

Debbie had already solved part of this problem by having her team pack most of their equipment in small satchels before they even arrived at the scene. I would later find out that she had roots in East Texas and wasn't exactly a stranger to the dense piney woods.

Scales suggested that they make the trip on four-wheelers. Calls immediately went out on the radio in an attempt to locate enough four-wheelers to accommodate the FBI team, as well as my father and myself.

While we were waiting for the four-wheelers to arrive, we got word that another crewmember had been found about five miles on the other side of Hemphill. At first they decided we would split up, half of the team staying here while the other half went across town to the other site. My father would stay with this group. The second group would drop me off at the funeral home so I could pick up the hearse and follow them out to the scene. After some discussion, the plan was changed to simply working the scenes one at a time. We would take care of this one, then proceed to the second site on the way through to Lufkin, much like we had on the first day.

In the meantime, three pickups with four-wheelers in their beds pulled up. I recognized two of the pickups; one belonged to Jason Pearson and another to Todd Parrish. Charlie and Tammy Waldrop set out ahead of us on their own four-wheeler while the members of the recovery team climbed on the newly arrived ones. Dad and I climbed into the Excursion. We would take it as far as it would go before we hopped on the back of a four-wheeler.

Dad laughed and nodded toward Debbie as she climbed on her own four-wheeler, then promptly asked us how it worked. Much to our surprise she managed like a pro as soon as she found the throttle.

The four-wheelers took the lead with the county patrol car behind them. The Excursion brought up the rear. We returned onto Fire Tower Road and made a left turn. Just before reaching the old fire tower, we took a fork to the right. A little farther along we stopped where a trail crossed the road. My father and I got out and started looking for rides.

Dad, of course, asked to ride with Debbie. I rolled my eyes.

When we started into the woods, Chad Murray took the lead, with the man in the NASA uniform riding behind him. Jason came second, with me perched behind him, sitting on top of the folded jump cot and the body bag. Brother Fred Raney drove the third four-wheeler with an agent riding behind him. Next came Debbie and another agent. Dad, having lost his bid to ride with Debbie, was bringing up the rear, riding on the back of a four-wheeler driven by another one of the agents.

We moved down the trail at what most people would consider a relatively easy pace. However, most people have never had to ride on the back of a four-wheeler while sitting on top of a jump cot and a slick rubber body bag. The only portion of my body that was actually touching the vehicle was my feet, and they were sharing the footrests with Jason. Every time we hit a bump, I bounced to one side or the other. I just knew I was going to topple off and get run over by Fred, who wasn't exactly an experienced four-wheeler operator.

On down the trail we discovered why Charlie and Tammy had gone ahead of us. They were using a chainsaw to clear out trees that had fallen in the path, so we wouldn't have to go around them like they had been doing all morning. We stopped and waited while they dragged one of the fallen trees out of the way.

Not much farther along we entered Seven Canyons, a little known, beautiful spot near the border of the National Forest. The deep wash is quite steep in most places, but the path we were following was accessible to off-road vehicles. The bouncing increased. I held on as we went into the canyon, crossed the meandering creek, and then back up the other side.

It was only a few hundred yards past this spot that we came up on a Game Warden's four-wheel drive pickup parked in the middle of the trail. I recognized one of our local Game Wardens, Henry Alvarez. We all parked our four-wheelers and Dad was the first one to ask the question that had to be on everyone's mind, "How'd you get that thing back here?"

Henry shrugged. "It wasn't hard, really."

We then heard something coming up the road behind us and turned to see Todd Parrish in his little blue pickup. The arrival of this second vehicle ruined any dramatic feeling I might have felt at our rugged four-wheeler trek into the wilderness.

After everyone had unloaded, the game wardens pointed us in the direction of the most recent site. Jason stayed behind with the game wardens while my father and I headed into the woods with the recovery team. Debbie had been right, the underbrush wasn't thick at all in this part of the woods. Terry left the site to meet us halfway and lead us in.

Before we set down our supplies and got to work, I took a long look at my surroundings. The astronaut had landed perfectly on top of a small mound on the side of a rolling, wooded hill, sort of a small false peak before the hill reached its actual summit. The hill descended gently to a small valley, and then dropped abruptly several yards away as it gave way to the green canyons. The lack of underbrush, combined with the sunlight beaming in from the perfectly clear day gave this site an idyllic feel. For a brief moment the beauty of the scene overwhelmed the tragedy. I found myself thinking that if not for the tragic circumstances, this might well be the perfect place to return to earth.

We lowered our heads as Brother Raney stepped forward and said his brief prayer.

When he was finished, we got to work making the recovery. My father and I stepped back while the FBI team photographed the site. After the pictures were taken and the GPS coordinates were recorded, I opened the body bag and stretched it out alongside the crewmember. Dad made sure that Marc, Debbie, and Terry were all satisfied with the site before we carefully placed the astronaut in the body bag. We then zipped the bag and loaded it onto the jump cot. My father and Terry got on either side of the front, Marc and I took the rear, and we walked the short distance back to the four-wheelers.

As we approached, Dad asked Henry if he could carry the cot and a couple of riders in the back of the truck without throwing us out. Henry said he could. We loaded the cot into the bed of the pickup, along with the four men who had been carrying the load. A young Asian-American agent from Debbie's team climbed into the back as well. He explained that a member of the recovery team was assigned to each piece of evidence, and he had been assigned to this one. He introduced himself as Tan Wen, and we welcomed him aboard.

Marc and Dad sat on one side of the stretcher, with Terry, Tan and myself on the other. I was crowded almost to the tailgate, which remained open due to the length of the jump cot. The ride out proved much easier than the ride in. The only point of excitement was in crossing the creek—the pickup had to build up speed to make sure it crossed without getting stuck. When we reached the other side of Seven Canyons, the road became quite smooth. We talked among ourselves, and for the first time it was just idle small talk, not operational plans on how to go about the recoveries.

Once we reached the dirt road, the jump cot was taken out of the truck and loaded into the back of the Excursion. The longer portion of the backseat was down to accompany the cot, but the shorter end was left up, allowing for a third rider, who I assumed would be Tan. However, he informed me that he would be riding behind us in a vehicle with the rest of his team, so, for once, I wasn't left searching for a ride. I hopped into the back of the Excursion. We got underway, heading for our second recovery of the day.

* * *

We returned to Charlie's place so the agents could get their cars. While we were there, we were given the exact location of the next site over the phone so we wouldn't have to talk on the radio. The next site was down Housen Hollow Road, less than a mile from Bob White's house. Sheriff Maddox and a Texas

Ranger were already at the site waiting on us.

We returned down Fire Tower Road, and then turned onto Highway 87 and headed toward town. Chad's county car was the only patrol car in our four-car convoy. We passed through Hemphill without any of the numerous reporters scattered about the town giving us a second glance.

* * *

We pulled barely a quarter of a mile down the muddy road before coming to a group of cars. Sheriff Maddox was in the middle of the road waiting on us. This was our site.

There wasn't much room for parking. The short driveway leading to the house on the left of the road was already filled, but there was another short road leading to an old garage to the right. Dad pulled into this road and one of the FBI's unmarked cars pulled in beside him. The other cars parked on the road, partially in the ditch.

As soon as they were out of the vehicles Dad and Tan discussed the crewmember in the Excursion. Dad offered to leave me to watch the car if Tan needed to be with his team. Tan replied that he had to stay with the body at all times. Dad took the keys out of his pocket, made a few jokes about Tan taking care of his vehicle before handing them to Tan, who gave a mock salute before taking the keys. Although we were only around him for a few hours, it was easy to see that Tan was a very likeable fellow.

When Dad and I started across the road to join the rest of the team, we were approached by a vaguely familiar person. This slender black-haired young man pulled out a notepad and asked if we could confirm or deny that another crewmember had been found. As soon as he spoke, I recognized him as the reporter who had tried to get an interview with me the previous afternoon while I was closing the funeral home.

"No comment," my father replied.

"Well, the fact that you're here says they've found something, doesn't it? You are John Starr, right?"

"No comment," Dad repeated, stepping around him.

Sheriff Maddox was already on his way over from across the road. "You need to get back up the road," he told the reporter as he approached.

The reporter turned to Maddox and gave a brief speech on his rights and the fact that this was a public road.

This didn't faze the sheriff in the least. "You can get back up the road right now, or I'll put you in the back of a patrol car and take you there."

Dad and I took our leave of the reporter and started across the road. We walked around to the back of the house, but found that while Dad and I were parking and dealing with the reporter, Terry, Marc, and Fred had been taken back to the site by the couple who had found the body. We were left without a scout to guide us to the site. We tried to find someone who could show us the way back, but no one left at the house had been to the site. However, the trail seemed obvious to me. Unlike the last site, the underbrush here was very dense. It was easy to tell where a person could and couldn't go.

Or so I thought.

"I think I can find it," I said, and, without waiting for an answer, I set out with the FBI team behind me and Dad bringing up the rear.

The first portion of our trek was very easy. It was a well-beaten path, easy to follow. In fact, I couldn't understand why no one else had volunteered to lead us—this was a breeze. About a hundred yards into the woods the trail began to narrow, but I was still confident I could follow the path. A little farther and we came to a narrow stream. On the other side, the trail ceased to exist. Across the stream, I thought I could see where the underbrush had been beaten down by the passage of the people before us, so I pressed on.

After my father crossed the stream, he called out, "Who's leading us anyway?"

"Byron," someone answered.

"Oh, God. We're lost."

"He says he knows where he's going," I heard Debbie reply.

"He's lying," Dad said, partially pulling my leg and partially concerned that I really was getting us lost. The agents might have been following me under the assumption that I knew this part of the woods, but Dad knew full well that I'd never been here in my life.

In truth, I really was beginning to think I might have missed the trail. I was right on the verge of swallowing my pride and suggesting we backtrack when the woods opened up into a muddy stream. I could see several footprints in the mud following the stream as it made its way through the woods. Apparently, we were still on the right track. The soupy stream was more mud than it was water, so when I took my first step my foot sank all the way to my ankle. I pulled my foot out for another step and almost lost my shoe in the process.

After getting to the other side of the stream, I took a brief look at the surrounding woods. I didn't catch any glimpse of color that would give away the group at the site, but I did see where the stream rounded off, curving to the left in the distance. I knew my dress shoes weren't made for walking in mud, so, rather than following the stream, I set off into the brush, trying to make a straight path through the woods where I could meet up with the stream at a later point.

Still under the assumption that I knew what I was doing, the recovery team followed right along without a word. My father, on the other hand, began questioning my abilities as a pathfinder as soon as he left the muddy creek and entered the woods.

Since we were no longer on the beaten path, we began to encounter thicker underbrush. I tore my suit twice and began to wish I'd stuck to the stream. I also became concerned that the path we were supposed to be following might only follow the stream for a short distance before heading into the woods again. If this was the case, I might miss the path altogether.

When I reached the stream I was much relieved to find the footprints still there. However, as I tried to take my first step out of the thicket and into the stream, I became tangled in a web of briars. While I was trying to pull free, the agent who had been following directly behind me stepped past me and into the stream. Much to my amusement, he promptly turned right and headed the wrong way. At least I wasn't the only one with a bad sense of direction. When one of the agents redirected him, my father overheard this and said, "I told you he'd get us lost."

From here on out we followed the stream and I didn't try any more shortcuts. It wasn't much farther before I saw NASA blue among the browns and greens of the thicket.

We had found the site.

* * *

We were still several yards away from the site when someone motioned for us to be quiet. They were praying. We stopped and lowered our heads. After Fred finished his prayer, we continued through the woods toward the site.

Two astronauts I'd never met were at the site along with Terry, Fred, and Marc, as were Herbert and Amber Welch, the couple who found the crewmember. Once again the FBI team photographed the site and the surrounding area, and then took the GPS coordinates. When they were finished my father and I once again assisted in placing the crewmember into the body bag.

If the walk into the woods had been difficult, it was going to be even harder walking out while carrying a body bag. To make matters worse, the jump cot was unavailable, being back at the Excursion, under the other crewmember. The heavy-duty body bags we use have six handles, one on each corner and two in the middle, but the trail we were on was too narrow to utilize the side straps. Terry and one of the astronauts got on the front, while one of the agents and I grabbed the straps in the rear. The rest of the agents went ahead to hold brush out of the way. We returned to the muddy stream, where I had considerable difficulty keeping my shoes on as we walked through the muck.

"See, this is why I took that shortcut through the woods," I grumbled to no one in particular.

"Oh, a little mud never hurt anyone," Debbie replied.

After we crossed to the second, not-so-muddy stream, a DPS officer came up the trail to meet us. The path was wider here, so I moved up to the middle strap and let him carry the rear, while another agent grabbed the middle strap on the other side.

We stopped near the edge of the woods. With the one exception, the site had been clear of reporters and had remained that way while we were in the woods. However, they still didn't want to walk the body bag out in full view of the small crowd of locals that had gathered at the Welch's house. Dad and one of the astronauts went ahead to see if they could back the Excursion behind the house.

After moving several cars out of the driveway, the Excursion was carefully backed into the muddy backyard and up to the edge of the woods. I climbed in the back and pulled the crewmember into the back until it was alongside the other crewmember on the jump cot.

When I got out of the Excursion, Dad and the astronauts were discussing a third site, this one a crew-related site in San Augustine County. They wanted us to make this recovery en route to Lufkin with the two crewmembers already recovered. A main concern was now daylight. The sun was rapidly setting behind the trees and by the time we would get to San Augustine it would be dark. However, they were told that the new site was close to a road. The recovery wouldn't take nearly as long as the other two.

Dad pointed out that we didn't have any more body bags with us. There were two more, but they were back at the funeral home. I offered to go get the body bags and meet them at the site if they would just find me a ride back to the funeral home. Texas Ranger Tom Young overheard this and offered to take me to town. One of the DPS officers then started giving us directions to the site. Dad knew that area well enough from when he used to run ambulances, but I didn't know my way around San Augustine County. This problem was solved when Tom said he knew where they were talking about. He offered to take me to get the body bags, and then take me out to the third scene.

We were burning precious daylight, so little time was wasted getting to Tom's car, and a considerable amount of lead was applied to the pedal on the way back into town. However, when we arrived at the funeral home, we were told that our trip to San Augustine had been called off. Apparently a body bag had been supplied by Wyman-Roberts Funeral Home in San Augustine. I thanked Tom for the ride and then returned to the funeral home, hoping to close and get home for some much needed rest.

* * *

I wasn't able to go straight home. Earlier in the day we had ordered some supplies from Dodge, our embalmer's supply company. Our sales rep had someone who not only wanted to drive all the way to Hemphill in order to get the order to us, but who also wanted to stay and help with the search. I appreciated the offer for help, but right then I just wanted to go home and climb in bed. However, I stayed around until Nate arrived.

Nate was given a brief tour of the funeral home, and then I ran up to the command post to drop off some supplies I had ordered for the FBI team. When Dad returned from Lufkin, he offered Nate a spare bed at Grandmaw's, which was where Dad was staying at the time.

7

The Media

W HEN I FINALLY arrived home Sunday, my wife Shelly met me at the door, excited about the fact that she had just heard on the news that all seven astronauts had been recovered.

"No, we've only located three so far," I replied, taking off my muddy dress shoes at the front door.

"They just said they've got all seven on the news. Maybe they found the other four in San Augustine or Nacogdoches."

"The only bodies have come out of Sabine County," I replied, as I walked through the living room on my way to take a much needed shower.

"Byron, I heard it on CNN."

"Then CNN's wrong."

When I got out of the shower, Shelly told me that CNN had retracted the statement. This was the first time I realized just how isolated this recovery operation was from the outside world.

A week later, while I was making a transportation run from Hemphill to Dr. Bruce's lab in Lufkin, the subject of the media came up in a conversation with the astronaut making the trip with me, Nancy Currie. She mentioned that the combined law enforcement branches in Sabine County were doing an outstanding job of handling the media. She had yet to be hassled by the customary packs of cameras, and she hadn't seen a single camera or reporter at a sensitive recovery site.

In truth, although diligence on the part of the officers

involved played a large part in how well the media was handled, there were other reasons which may have played an even larger role.

Probably the single most important factor in controlling the media was the regular media briefings. These briefings were held two times a day, starting on Sunday. During the first week, Co-Incident Commanders Tom Maddox and Billy Ted Smith kept the media abreast of the situation, giving enough information to keep the media from grasping at straws, while holding back any information that might compromise the operation.

Of course, the competitive nature of journalism will always push some reporters to dig deeper for that extra bit of information not available from normal outlets. However, one of the greatest barriers to this form of investigative journalism proved to be the people of Sabine County. For the most part, the people were polite and friendly and in many cases genuinely fond of the reporters who were visiting the area during this time. Many of the locals freely gave interviews and expressed their opinions on the operation. However, the people of Sabine County took great pride in this operation right from the beginning, and anyone who found themselves privy to inside information was very unlikely to give this information to an outsider. The three shuttle crewmembers who were found on the first two days were located by locals who were not involved in the recovery operation, but instead of calling the media, they called the authorities. They didn't get to see their names in the papers or their faces on the news, but they were rewarded with the knowledge that they had helped in the honorable and respectful recovery of the newest heroes of two nations.

It is also worth mentioning that the only time the reporters reached a sensitive crew-related site was before the wagons of the search effort had been circled. If the discovery in Bob White's pasture had been made the following day, or even later in the afternoon, more than likely the media would not have found out about this site.

Another reason the media was much easier to handle

than expected was the two cities of Lufkin and Nacogdoches. While the astronauts were being recovered in Sabine County, the outside focus on the operation was directed more toward these two areas than anywhere else. The search and recovery operations in Sabine County were controlled out of Hemphill's Incident Command Post; however, the overall command center for the entire operation was based in Lufkin. Also, the media turned their attention elsewhere simply because of the fact that we didn't have room to accommodate reporters in Sabine County. There was only one motel in the county and it had filled on the first night of the accident. Many of the reporters found hotel rooms in Lufkin and Nacogdoches.

This made sense on many different levels. While the astronauts were found in Sabine County, more of the shuttle itself was found in Nacogdoches County than in any other area, and Lufkin command was doing an excellent job with its major press conferences. And while Lufkin and Nacogdoches are only twenty miles apart, Hemphill is a good sixty-five miles from either of these two cities. Rather than lug their equipment back and forth between the two areas, many reporters chose to stay in one place, or perhaps visit Sabine County only once or twice, then report "live" from Nacogdoches. At one point, my wife saw a newscast in which the reporter said he was reporting live from Hemphill, Texas, with the Nacogdoches County Courthouse clearly visible in the background.

Another very important factor in the successful handling of the media was the attitude of the reporters themselves. I had a chance to get a close up look at the media in action during the two weeks that I was involved in the recovery operation. As a rule they were friendly, polite, and, while they were certainly eager, they usually stopped well short of being pushy.

During the opening stages of the operation, Billy Ted Smith served as Co-Incident Commander, as well as Information Officer. He later remarked that he developed close working relations with several individuals in the media, particularly Maria Hinojosa of CNN. He recalled that by the end of his one-week stint as Information Officer he could actually give Maria information and tell her it was off the record, and this information would never reach the public.

Halfway through the first week of the operation, the U.S. Forest Service started handling the news briefings. During their first briefing, Greg was asked if there had been any progress in the search for the remaining crew members; Greg Cohrs informed them that he couldn't answer specific questions concerning the search for the crew. Much to his surprise, not only did the reporters instantly drop the subject, but it wasn't even brought up in the briefing on the following day.

Still, there was a definite "us versus them" mentality on both sides of the yellow tape. The officers who were used to watch the entrance to the command center and to keep the press on the other side of the line could have certainly been put to better use walking the woods. And I'm sure there are those among the media who felt that if they had been supplied with a little more information, they wouldn't have been left stumbling along in the dark so often.

* * *

There were some instances in which the media did get a little overzealous, especially during the first few days. At times this frantic behavior was quite humorous to the laid back rural folk. Throughout the operation the reporters were kept out of both the Incident Command Post and the Volunteer Staging Area. However, they lurked outside both of these places trying to interview the workers and volunteers as they would come and go.

With only a pair of two-seater restrooms, the VFW hall didn't exactly have sufficient facilities for the mass of volunteers who converged on the Staging Area. Port-o-potties were on the way, but for the first couple of days the volunteers had to make do. As a result, a line often formed outside the restrooms. In true country fashion, the local searchers would quite often walk across the road to the woods and relieve themselves behind a tree. On the second day of the operation, a local gentleman, who wished to remain anonymous, set foot in the woods for that very reason. However, while searching for a suitable tree, he found a rather large piece of the shuttle. Still sporting a full bladder, he returned to the VFW Post and reported what he had found. A group from the Forest Service took over from there and went into the woods to mark the debris and get the GPS coordinates.

There was still a line at the restroom, and the volunteer still needed to find a tree. However, the reporters had been watching when he stepped into the woods and they saw him when he came back to the VFW hall to contact the authorities. When he returned to the woods, they assumed he was involved in searching that area, so a small group followed him. Before he reached the edge of the woods, the volunteer noticed he was being followed. He stopped and answered a few questions, and tried to tell the reporters that he wasn't searching the woods. Since there were ladies present and cameras rolling, this country gentleman didn't want to tell them what he was really doing. The reporters were used to people trying to tell them they weren't involved when they really were, so, since he wasn't exactly offering up an alibi, they obviously thought he was lying.

Finally, he was able to convince the reporters that he had just stumbled on the debris and wasn't currently involved in an organized search of the area. However, when he was finally able to slip away into the woods, they followed him anyway. Since this guy had apparently located debris just by walking in the woods, the reporters suddenly decided that's what they wanted to do. They hit the woods across from the VFW hall with all the enthusiasm of a kindergarten class on an Easter egg hunt. Now the poor guy was having to dodge the amateur searchers, while still carrying on his own search for a little privacy. It took quite some time for the poor gentleman to find a tree that didn't have a reporter snooping around it, but eventually he did.

Another incident occurred one day when USFS Ranger

Marcus Beard was on his way across the street to the Command Post following the media briefing. The media wasn't allowed inside the yellow line, but anything outside of the line was fair game. They recognized Marcus and immediately swarmed him, blocking his path and barraging him with questions. The questions had no more than begun than a State Trooper waded through the reporters and firmly grasped Marcus by the upper arm. "Sir, you need to come with me," the trooper barked.

Even as they walked through the reporters, the officer maintained his grip on Marcus's arm. The Ranger was now convinced he was in trouble for something, although he couldn't imagine what. "Am I being arrested?" Marcus asked, half jokingly.

"No," the trooper said, loosening his grip. "You just looked like you needed a little help."

Marcus laughed and asked, "Can you be here at the same time tomorrow?"

"No problem."

* * *

The main conflict of interest between the operation and the media centered around what the press calls "the public's right to know" and the astronauts' families' right to privacy. Yes, the public was honestly concerned, and they wanted to know how the recovery was progressing. However, the families needed to find out about the progress of the search through the proper channels, not through the media. It appears that this portion of the operation was every bit as successful as the rest.

8

The Nose Cone and the Space Monkeys

ON THE MORNING the shuttle crashed, Nathan Ener and his friend, Tim "Peewee" Mitchell, had been putting the finishing touches on the fence in front of Nathan's house. They were in the process of running wire to the two lamps flanking his drive when the terrible rumbling noise tore their attention from their work. The sound seemed to come from behind Nathan's house, leading him to believe that a dozer had been working in the woods and had slipped a track. Little did they know that a major portion of the shuttle had passed almost directly overhead, striking across the road in the woods.

On the way back to his house to rest his weary legs, Nathan discovered a large piece of off-white material. As he was investigating this discovery, he noticed another piece of material a few feet away. The second piece was similar in size—a little more than a foot across—but it was much darker, and this grayish piece of cloth gave of a foul chemical odor. A few feet further, Nathan found yet another piece of strange cloth, this one similar to the first. Not sure of what he had found, Nathan gathered the pieces and took them to his shed before returning to the house.

Once inside, Nathan's wife informed him that the Space Shuttle Columbia had fallen apart upon reentry and scattered debris along a narrow corridor through East Texas. Nathan immediately returned to the shed for the pieces of material. He placed them exactly as he had found them, then called the sheriff's department. Nathan spent the next day riding the roads on his Polaris buggy. He didn't even have to get off the road to assist in the search; debris was everywhere. He found several pieces either lying by the roadside or not far off the road, including a metal ring that measured eight feet in diameter.

Late Sunday afternoon, Nathan took the time to search some of the areas near his house. While driving through a neighboring pasture, he found several smaller pieces of debris. These new discoveries, combined with the material found the day before, roused his curiosity as to what might be in the woods near his home. However, it was getting late, so he would have to wait until the next morning.

* * *

Searching the swampy and densely wooded area around Nathan's house wouldn't be easy, especially on a pair of bad knees. Luckily, Peewee Mitchell returned to the house that morning to assist in the search. First, they walked the area behind the house, the direction from which the sound had seemed to come. This turned up several small pieces of debris, but no major finds. After searching behind the house, the two men turned their attention to the area immediately around the house. Finding nothing new, they moved on to the marshy woods across the road.

Nathan Ener's house was located on a small dirt road called Bayou Bend, located just outside of Hemphill. The road is nothing more than a little loop that leaves Highway 83 at an angle, then travels in a short semicircle for less than a quarter of a mile before once again joining the highway. About half of the land between Bayou Bend and Highway 83 is marshy, while the other half is somewhat higher ground and only swampy during wet spells.

Nathan and Peewee split up. Nathan set out straight across from his house. This would put him in the swampiest portion of the woods, but would make his search somewhat shorter. Peewee went into the woods a hundred yards or so farther down.

After about an hour of fruitless search, the two men returned to the house and met at the gate.

"Find anything?" Peewee asked.

"No. How about you?"

"Nothing. There might be something in that old dump site, though."

"Dump site? There's not a dump over there."

"There's not?"

Nathan followed as Peewee retraced his steps into the woods. Before they even reached the site, Nathan began to notice several limbs and even a few treetops broken overhead. Barely one-hundred yards off Bayou Bend, they found Peewee's so-called dump site. A large piece of metal had ripped through the trees and slammed into the earth, creating a crater that was roughly twenty foot in diameter and a tall embankment opposite the hole. Shards of metal were embedded deep into several of the trees along the embankment side of the crater.

Nathan stepped to the edge of the wreckage. Everything was twisted out of shape, but it otherwise seemed polished and clean, rather than burned as he had expected. At the center of the twisted metal, he found a fractured charcoal colored dome, partially buried in the ground. It was the shuttle's nose cone.

He looked back in the direction of his home. The tall pines hid his house from sight, but he knew the approximate location of his home. It was easy to tell from the path the debris had made through the trees that he was lucky his house hadn't been hit. In fact, we were all lucky, since not a single person was struck and only two houses in Sabine County were hit—and those were struck with relatively minor pieces of debris.

As soon as he returned home, Nathan contacted the authorities. As it turned out, the importance of the find was not realized at first. Nathan's report was registered as a standard debris report, and debris reports were being answered in the order they were received.

The next day Nathan called again. This time he was more specific about his find.

Within a few hours Bayou Bend was blocked off on both ends while a swarm of FBI agents, EPA officers and workers, and NASA officials converged on the site. The ever-present reporters also converged at the barricaded ends of the road.

* * *

While the various organizations started to work removing the nose cone, Nathan continued his independent search elsewhere. Tuesday afternoon Nathan was joined by Steve Arney, who closed the doors on his concrete business for two weeks in order to search for debris. He and Steve used Nathan's buggy to help them search along the roadsides.

The two men would be up well before sunrise and wouldn't return until after sunset. At first they would report everything they found to the authorities as soon as they found it, but their efforts proved to be so successful that the command finally just gave them their own spool of marking ribbon and told them to mark everything they found and not to bother calling it in until they returned in the afternoon.

Of course, if the two-man search team found something significant, they weren't about to let it wait until they returned home at dark. At one point they found and reported an item that the command thought might have been part of the shuttle's cabin. An official from NASA, three FBI agents, and a German Shepherd trained to locate bodies were all packed into the buggy with Nathan and Steve, neither of whom were exactly what one would call small men.

As the buggy topped a small rise, Nathan pointed out an adjacent hill and explained that this was where they were going. When Nathan turned in order to take a longer route around an area of heavy brush between the two rises, one of the agents asked why they didn't just go through the brush.

"That's a thicket," Steve replied, nodding toward the tangled vines.

"I'll bet this thing could make it."

"Those are saw-briars. Do you know what saw-briars are?"

"Stickers."

Steve sighed and shook his head. "Where are you from?"

"New York."

"That explains it."

When they reached the site, Steve got off the buggy and walked over to the thicket. While the FBI team was investigating the site, he took out his pocket knife, cut off a saw-briar vine, and returned to the group. He presented the vine to the agent and asked, "Do these look like stickers to you?"

The agent looked over the vine and its thorns, which were over an inch long. "I guess not." Then the agent laughed. "I'm going to have to take this back home with me. They'll never believe it if I don't bring proof."

* * *

During another trip to a site, a genuine Sabine County legend was born. The buggy was not quite as crowded this time around—they were less one man and the dog. On board Nathan's buggy this time were one NASA official, two men with Texas Parks and Wildlife, and Nathan and Steve. One of the two men with the Texas Parks and Wildlife was Lin Marcantel, a life-long resident of Sabine County; the other was a young biologist.

When the group stopped at the site, Steve got off the buggy and started searching the ground. He found several round rabbit droppings and placed them on a large leaf. Steve mentioned to Nathan that they should try to convince the young man that the droppings came from something out of the shuttle, but Steve never realized how far his friend was going to take the matter. Nathan called Lin and the man from NASA over and told them the plan. They both thought it was hilarious, but all agreed that Nathan should do the talking.

The young man noticed that he was being left out of the conversation and came over and asked what they were talking about.

Nathan gave the man from NASA a grave look and asked, "Should we tell him?"

"Yes, I think he needs to know."

Nathan then commenced with a tall tale about a group of monkeys that had been on board the shuttle. He told how the military had paid NASA to test chemical and biological agents on these monkeys. The story ended with the revelation that these monkeys would be incredibly dangerous if they were still alive.

Lin and the NASA official were unable to talk for fear that they would burst into laughter the moment they opened their mouths, and Steve wasn't even able to look at the young man.

Nathan rose from his seat and led the way over to Steve's pile of rabbit pellets. He pointed to the pile and said, "And now we have evidence that the monkeys might have survived the crash."

The young biologist leaned down for a closer look.

"Don't touch it!" Nathan snapped, "That's evidence!"

The young man carefully folded his hands behind his back, as if they might betray him and accidentally brush against the space monkey poop.

And this was only the first of several tales involving Nathan's space monkeys. As the operation pushed on into the second week, these two men became favorites of the government officials and the reporters alike. Outgoing and always looking for a laugh, Nathan spun tall tales to the gullible about the experimental monkeys that had survived Columbia's crash and were now running amuck through the woods. From NASA personnel on down to the common searcher, everyone who saw Nathan and Steve would ask how the search for the monkeys was going. And Nathan's tales grew wilder with each passing day, reaching a climax when he claimed to have been chased out of the woods by a one-armed monkey carrying a syringe.

At one point Nathan took out an ad in the Sabine County Reporter enquiring about monkey traps, monkey feed, and tranquilizer darts. He slyly mentioned that anyone with information should contact him or Steve, but, since his phone was unlisted, Steve, who didn't even know about the ad, received all the calls. The next day Steve was getting calls from all over the county. The local grocery store even called and offered to send over a crate of bananas.

Steve often found himself embarrassed by his friend's antics. He feared that someone might take offense at his friend's tall tales, thinking that Nathan was poking fun at the tragedy. In truth, Nathan's humorous stories provided an escape from the stress of the operation. Surrounded by such tragedy, the workers and volunteers needed something to laugh about—and Nathan Ener's space monkeys fit the bill perfectly.

9

Walking the Woods

WHEN FRED RANEY gave his Monday morning prayer at the Volunteer Staging Area, it was a little different than before. This morning's prayer was Joshua 1:6-9. These were the same verses read by Commander Husband just before Columbia lifted off on her fateful journey. Every morning over the next few weeks, Fred would read these words from the Old Testament to the assembled volunteers, not just in honor of our six American astronauts, but also out of respect for Israeli astronaut Ilan Ramon.

Once again, the Sabine County volunteers prepared a massive breakfast. They continued preparing and serving the food while assembled volunteers ate. As the search volunteers began finishing their breakfasts, the kitchen volunteers started cleaning and preparing to make the lunches that would be taken out into the field.

Some of Sunday's searchers had failed to return for the second day. Quite a few had to return to their jobs once the weekend was over, a few of the younger volunteers had to go back to school, and some had simply found that they weren't cut out for trampling through dense underbrush from sunup to sundown. Despite this, there was actually a slight increase in the number of volunteers. Quite a few people had come to the VFW hall who hadn't known about Sunday's search, and volunteers from other counties were now beginning to arrive.

The National Guard had also arrived with some 150 soldiers to assist in the search. This influx of personnel was greatly appreciated, but there were rumors circulating that once enough soldiers arrived, the volunteers would be sent home. Just as the operation leaders were dreading the possibility of the military taking over the operation, the local volunteers weren't happy with the prospect of outsiders taking over the search operation. As tired as they were from the first day's search, this was their county and this was their mission. They wanted to see this job through to the end.

* * *

Several changes were made after the first day of organized searching. For one thing, the volunteer groups serving in the area were now divided into six groups instead of four. Randy Perwitt and Debbie Casto were placed in command of the new groups. On Sunday afternoon, eighteen additional U. S. Forest Service officials had arrived from the Kisatchie National Forest in Louisiana. Greg decided to divide these newcomers up into each of the six groups in order to address various skills levels and also allow the newcomers to work with people with local knowledge.

The National Guard units were deployed in three groups of about fifty each. They were sent to the Bronson area, where they would push toward Highway 96. Yesterday's four Forest Service led groups were deployed on either side of the searched area on Farm Road 2024; they were to search in both directions along the corridor, with two teams traveling southeast and two traveling northwest. The two new teams were deployed near Beckham Road, where they began working their way northwest.

* * *

It was raining lightly when the volunteers made their way out of the VFW hall and began loading into the buses. Today they were making the move from the hall to the buses a good hour earlier than the day before. After they were loaded, however, the buses were cranked, but left idling for the better part of an hour. After a while, the diesel fumes became too thick in the bus, so Bob and several other volunteers left their seats and stepped outside into the rain to get some fresh air. The impatient searchers grumbled at the delay, but the search team leaders knew that the operation's planners were busily working out the final details of today's search.

It was still several minutes before the volunteers were loaded back into the buses and taken to the second day's drop off point. Once they were there, the improvements from the day before became readily apparent. Although the Forest Service was in charge of the groups, Bob's position as the fire chief placed him in a bit of an unofficial command role. He was to walk behind and help keep his subsection of the line as straight and orderly as possible.

There was also a noticeable improvement in the overall preparation of the individual searchers. In order to keep Sunday's cramps from making an unwanted return visit, Bob had eaten an orange at breakfast and was carrying an orange with him for lunch. Apparently he wasn't the only person who had been given this handy bit of information, since he noticed several other volunteers carrying oranges with them. Other important supplies had begun to make their appearance—walking sticks and machetes were common items, and everyone was carrying a tremendous amount of water. Todd Parrish was almost comically weighted down with precious H^2O, carrying several canteens of water in his belt and a flask in each sock.

This extra preparation proved to be a godsend, because Monday was even more difficult than the day before. Much of the privately owned search area covered had been clear-cut a few years before and now contained five to ten years growth, making the area extremely thick with undergrowth and brush. Once again they struggled their way through the dense vegetation, locating and marking pieces of shuttle debris as they went.

At noon the Red Cross once again brought rations and water out to the volunteers. Although most of the volunteers had brought their own supplies today, it was impossible to have too much water and food.

During this lull, Bob leaned up against a tree and began carefully peeling his orange. With his face and arms covered with scratches from the vines and his wildlands suit tattered and worn, he cut a rough image.

Todd was sprawled across the ground nearby, partaking of one of his many containers of water, when he paused, sat up, and affixed Bob with a peculiar stare.

Bob looked up from his orange. "What?"

"I was just thinking," Todd said. "I sure would've hated to tangle with you when you were thirty years old."

Of course, in terms of stamina, Todd could've done some boasting himself. Only a few months ago, he had been involved in a motorcycle accident that had seriously injured both of his legs. He had been in rehabilitation for several months and had actually been allowed to leave by default. One of the tests required him to step up on a block positioned several inches off the ground; this was resolved only after convincing the doctor that his inability to manage this particular obstacle had more to do with his short stature than his injuries. However, Todd was out there, trudging through terrain that was considerably more difficult than any rehabilitation obstacle course.

After the lunch break, the search line set out once more. By the end of the day, Bob's wildlands suit was in tattered ruins. He was utterly exhausted, but at least the oranges had warded off the leg cramps.

His flu seemed to be returning, and an important doctor's appointment would keep him away from the line Tuesday morning, but he would be back on Wednesday, if at all possible.

10

The Third Day's Recoveries

MY FATHER AND I were lucky in that there were very few deaths in the county while we were involved in the recovery effort. Monday morning was one of the few days in which we had a funeral service—I handled the service while Dad stayed at the office, ready to go at a moment's notice. Nate had reported to the Volunteer Staging Area early that morning. Jason came to work long enough to help me with the service. As soon as we were finished, he returned to the woods with the volunteers.

I returned from the graveside portion of the funeral at a little after noon. With everything quiet at work, we gathered in the front office and listened to the handheld police radio. There was still considerably more chatter than normal, but, since reports of newly-found debris had slowed down, the traffic on the radio had died down somewhat. We knew that any discovery of crewmembers or crew-related items would be kept off the air, but we hoped we could tell by the activity and the units responding to calls when we might be called out. Sure enough, around three o'clock several messages were sent from the field to the Incident Command Post. There was little doubt that the search teams had made an important discovery.

Dad made a phone call to the sheriff's office, but the sheriff was at the ICP and the dispatcher wasn't sure what had been found. We returned to listening to our makeshift scanner. The more we heard, the more we became convinced we would be getting a call at any minute.

Sure enough, at roughly half past three, we received a call from the Command Post. Dad and I hopped into the Excursion and headed to town.

Shane gave us directions as soon as we arrived. There had been another crew-related find down Houson Hollow Road. We were told to keep going past our last location; an officer would stop us on down the road, near the new site.

* * *

No one was waiting to flag us down when we reached our destination, but it was quite obvious we were where we were supposed to be by the number of cars in the area. There was a small open area in the woods to the left; this is where most of the cars were parked. A barbwire fence ran along the right of the road. Behind it was an open pasture surrounded by woods.

Fred Raney was at the scene, as was Roger McBride. However, the number of strange faces far outnumbered those I recognized. About a half-dozen FBI agents were milling around the vehicles. Apparently this was a different recovery team.

Dad found out which agent was in charge and asked how we could help. The agent said the body was across the pasture and deep into the woods; we were to stay on the road and they would bring the body to us, but Dad suggested we follow them as far as the back of the pasture. He explained that, while the Excursion wasn't a four-wheel drive, the sheriff's patrol pickup was. The cot could be loaded into the back of the pickup and taken across the pasture, cutting their walking distance in half. The agent agreed, so we loaded our jump cot and a pair of body bags into the back of the pickup. I climbed into the back with the equipment, while the recovery team began loading into a pair of vehicles for a trek into the muddy pasture. Roger and Fred got in the cab of the pickup and Dad climbed in the back with me.

We parked our vehicles on the top of a small rise, near the back of the pasture. I grabbed the jump cot and a box of gloves and asked if they would like for me to come along and lend a hand. I was told to remain where I was and they would let me know if I was needed. In fact, when Roger made the same offer, they didn't want him to come along either. I was a bit perplexed. Sure, they were a trained FBI team, but, the way I saw it, the ignorant locals they were leaving behind had performed four space shuttle recoveries; that was four more than these experts had performed.

I tossed the cot into the back of the pickup and asked Roger why we weren't allowed at this site.

"New team, new rules," Roger replied with a shrug.

* * *

We waited at the edge of the woods for about a half an hour before Roger received a call on the radio. They wanted him to turn on his sirens. Roger complied, letting his sirens howl for a few seconds before turning them off. A small herd of cows had just built up enough courage and curiosity to make it halfway across the pasture to investigate our presence. The sudden noise sent them thundering back to the far side of the field.

Still somewhat bitter at being left behind, I turned to Dad and muttered. "Don't tell me they're lost."

"Apparently someone is," Roger said from the pickup's cab.

I began scanning the edge of the woods in hope that I might see some movement or a patch of color that might give away the lost team. While I was keeping lookout, Roger was asked to turn the sirens on again.

Not long after Roger turned on his sirens a second time, a tall Jasper city Police officer in SWAT-type fatigues stepped out of the woods. He was coming from an entirely different direction than the one taken by the FBI team, so I didn't see him until he was in the pasture with us. Dad asked if he was the one who was lost. The officer turned out to be Mike Poindexter, Division Leader for Ground Search Groups 3 and 4. He said he wasn't lost. His groups were just finishing their day when he heard the sirens and, thinking it might be a distress call, he set off in our direction.

Mike took a long drink from his canteen, then proceeded to tell us about his day. This had been a rough day on the line.

A few minutes later Roger received another request that he turn on his sirens. Once again the brief yelp panicked the cows, sending them running back and forth along the far side of the pasture. A few more minutes passed and Roger received another request to turn on his sirens. This time they asked that he leave them on. Needless to say, the cows really freaked out this time. I thought they were going to tear down the opposite fence.

I left our small group and returned to the edge of the woods. This time, after a few minutes of scanning the woods, I saw someone moving in the trees. They were definitely headed our way. I told Roger I could see them, so he turned off his sirens.

Only two of the agents returned from the site. They mentioned that this was another significant find, and that they had returned because the astronaut at the scene had requested Brother Raney. Once again I offered to help, but they declined. I then offered them our jump cot. At first they declined this as well, but they took me up on the offer after I explained how much easier it would be to use the cot instead of carrying a body bag out.

Once again they disappeared into the woods, leaving us back at the vehicles. They were almost out of sight when Roger mentioned that Fred wasn't in the best of health and that he ought to go make sure he didn't overexert himself. When Roger set off after the group, it left only my father, Mike, and myself in the pasture.

I became restless and once again ventured to the edge of the woods. After a while I saw our group returning from the site. Two agents were walking ahead, pushing brush out of the way, while Roger, an astronaut and two agents carried the jump cot. One of the agents carrying the cot was Terry Lane. Apparently he and the astronaut had stayed at the site with the remains while the FBI team prepared for the recovery; this was why I hadn't seen him earlier. It was certainly apparent he had been out for some time; he was wringing with sweat.

I found a low place in the barbwire fence and directed them to it. When they reached the fence, I helped them over; then I took over for Roger and carried the cot the rest of the way to the pickup. Once the cot was loaded into the bed of the pickup, a member of the FBI recovery team, the astronaut, my father, and myself climbed in as well.

Before we got started, Terry spoke briefly to my father. Apparently, there was another crew-related find nearby. Darkness was rapidly approaching, so we would have to be quick. It's easy enough to become lost in the East Texas woods in the daylight; in the dark, it's almost impossible not to get turned around.

Roger drove the pickup back across the pasture. At the gate the Excursion was backed as far into the muddy pasture as we dared. The cot was taken from the back of the pickup and loaded into the Excursion.

Once again, I raised the partial seat in the back of the Excursion and offered my front seat to the astronaut. He declined, saying he would rather ride in the back.

* * *

So far the operation had been blessed with clear weather, but there had been enough rain the week before to turn Houson Hollow Road into a quagmire. In fact, the portion of the road ahead of us was in far worse shape than the pasture had been. Only two of the vehicles present had four-wheel drive, but, despite the condition of the road, Dad thought he could manage in the Excursion. The sheriff's patrol pickup, once again with Roger driving, took the lead, with the Excursion in the middle and an FBI blazer bringing up the rear.

The short drive to the next scene went well. There was no small amount of sliding and spinning, but we never came close to bogging down.

After a couple of miles of mud, we passed one logging road on our right. When we came to a second logging road, we turned. Before we turned in, I spotted a figure well on down the road running our way and waving for us to stop. It was Nate. I told Dad to stop. Apparently, Roger hadn't seen us stop; he kept going. Most logging roads are a straight shot to a logging site without any side roads or junctions, but we were still worried about being left behind just in case there was a junction or two; the only person who knew the location of the next site was in the car ahead of us. We took off after Roger. Luckily, Nate was able to run and catch the car behind us.

The patrol pickup stopped on down the road and we pulled in behind them. Everybody got out and started making preparations for another trip into the woods.

While the recovery team was getting ready, Roger received a call on the radio. Shane had been unable to contact Terry by his cell phone; he needed Terry to call in as soon as possible. Cellular reception in Sabine County has always been terrible. The additional towers brought in for the operation helped somewhat, but the county was still covered with dead spots. Terry checked his cell phone, and sure enough, he didn't have any reception. Brother Raney's phone, however, had just enough reception to make a call. Terry used Fred's phone and called the command center.

Apparently a third site had been discovered. Terry told them it would be some time before we were finished here. In fact, with nightfall rapidly approaching, it would probably be dark before we finished this recovery. Another recovery team would handle this third site and they would meet us at the Sheriff's Office, where we would transfer the remains to the Excursion for transportation.

When he got off the phone, Terry spoke with Dad about what he had discussed with Shane. Terry already knew Dad would do anything that was needed, but he asked for our assistance out of courtesy. Dad, of course, said he would help in any way he could.

When the FBI team got ready to go, I once again asked one of the agents with the recovery team if they needed help. Like the conversation between my father and Terry, I already knew the answer, but asked anyway out of courtesy. As usual, one agent was left behind with the body, as were Roger, my father, Nate, and myself.

While we were standing around, Nate asked the agent why we hadn't come on down to where he had been standing earlier. He had been on the search group that had discovered the site. Since he had experience in the funeral industry, he was left with the remains after the searchers moved on. While we were working on the first site, an agent had arrived and taken the GPS coordinates of the site. It was discovered that Housen Hollow Road passed within one-hundred yards of the site, almost five times closer than the path they had been taking from the logging road. Nate had been sent out to wave us to this shorter path, but when we saw him down the road, frantically waving at us, everyone assumed he was thumbing a ride. He said he mentioned the shortcut to the agents after we got out of the cars, but, since we were already here, they didn't seem interested. It was doubtful they realized just how much shorter the alternate path was.

Dad then spoke up and told the agent he thought everything would go smoother if the FBI would stick to one team. I winced when he said this, thinking the agent would take it as an insult. However, our new companion proved to be very open-minded. He agreed, for the most part, but, even though there were only seven astronauts to be recovered, the nature of the accident meant there would be more than seven crew-related recovery sites. One team could handle seven sites, but they would be stretched thin if they had to work a few dozen. It was a good point. So far we had only received calls on two or three sites at a time, but what would happen if we happened to receive calls on several at once?

It didn't take long for us to warm up to the agent who had been left behind. He was from a small town in Tennessee, so the transition to the piney woods of East Texas had come fairly easy. Although we hadn't been able to work directly with this

FBI team, talking to this team member made me feel better about today's recoveries. It was odd, they were the experts and I was just a small town undertaker, but I had felt as though I needed to be there to make sure everything was done properly; I had been angry at being left behind simply because I wanted to make sure everything was handled with care and not like a crime scene. Now I realized that this team was very professional, but not scientifically calloused. It also helped that Terry Lane was with them—I had the utmost respect for that man.

It was almost dark before the recovery team returned with the body bag stretched out between them, and night had fallen by the time we got back to Hemphill. We were instructed to back up to the covered sally port on the side of the law enforcement center. Once we were backed into place, a white cooler was placed in the back of the Excursion.

I waited while they arranged for an escort to Lufkin. After they left, I asked Roger to take me back to the funeral home.

11
Logistics and Communication

MARK ALLEN WAS a sergeant in the Patrol Division of the Jasper County Sheriff's Department, working out of Buna in the southern portion of the county. However, he also served as a deputy with the area's Emergency Management Corps. As a result he had been working the shuttle incident since day one. On the first two days, Mark had worked along Toledo Bend, assisting with the first loosely organized efforts to search the banks. He had helped pave the way for the newly created Water Search Branch, which was then under the direction of Jasper County Sheriff Billy Rowels.

On Monday, Co-Incident Commander Billy Ted Smith approached Mark with a new assignment. Billy wanted to utilize Mark's skills of organization in the crucial role of Logistics Section Chief.

When Mark took over the Logistics Section, the ball was already rolling thanks to the efforts of the Incident Commanders, their staff, the other Section Chiefs, Branch Directors, and the initial Logistics Chief, Janie Peveto. However, there was still much work to be done. Mark's primary task was to remove a thorn that had been in the side of the operation since day one— he had to do something about the poor communication. Close to fifty phone lines had already been installed at Incident Command Center, but more were needed. Mark contacted Valor Telecom and had them install twenty-five more lines. Throughout the next week, more lines would be ordered and installed, as every organization seemed to need multiple phone, computer, and fax lines. By the end of the second week, Mark had ordered over 200 phone lines installed in the Incident Command Post and the Volunteer Staging Area.

Mark then turned his attention to a much more pressing issue—communication in the field. Insufficient radio channels and the county's notoriously poor cellular reception had plagued the operation from the beginning. Mark called Verizon to see if they could help solve the problem. After playing phone tag for the better part of the afternoon, Mark finally found himself with a Verizon employee on the other end of the line who happened to be an ex-Army Ranger. This person certainly understood what communication meant to a command structure. Several free cell phones were sent overnight to the Incident Command Center, and several of the company's portable towers were on the way.

The use of Verizon's cell phones, equipment, and even free air time came with one small condition—they wanted public mention in one of the daily briefings. This wasn't a problem. The next morning, Billy Ted Smith thanked Verizon for their efforts. In fact, the public mention proved to be a wonderful idea. Not only did it serve as great advertisement for Verizon; it also brought in other cellular companies who didn't want to be left out of the act. Soon temporary cell towers from various companies sprang up all along the shuttle's path.

The second daunting task Mark faced was the health of the searchers. Working out in the cold, wet weather, many of the searchers were becoming ill. And the common cold was the least of their problems. With several hundred people eating in the same building and sharing the same restrooms, it came as no surprise when dysentery came on with a vengeance. By the Mark time took over the Logistics Section there had already been eighty reported cases of diarrhea.

Mark contacted KC Drugs in Hemphill and set up an account. He quickly drained the pharmacy of every stomach remedy that they could lay their hands on before moving on to the other local pharmacies. Once these supplies were depleted,

Mark moved on to the Wal-Mart Pharmacy in Jasper.

The two initial problems of communication and illness were the most significant faced by Mark in his two week tenure as the Logistics Chief, but his job was far from over. During the next couple of weeks the Logistics Section was constantly swamped with orders ranging from GPS tracking systems to thumbtacks. When the shuttle had fallen out of the sky, the weather had been warm and sunny, so most of the initial responders had arrived without the thick clothing or rain gear they would need. Miles of extension cord would be needed. Some organizations lacked office supplies. Fuel had to be brought in for the vehicles. The search teams needed compasses. Mark's shopping list was unending, and he spent hours on the telephone trying to tie down loose ends for the better part of the operation.

Mark wasn't alone, though. The day after he took over the lonely position of Logistics Chief, Greg Kelly, another member of the Emergency Management Corps, was assigned to the Logistics Section as Marc's deputy. Billy Lumpkin, of the U.S. Forest Service, and Howard Ure, of the Texas Forest Service, were also assigned to Mark's Section, and Belinda Gay was officially placed in charge of the Food Unit, although this was actually official recognition for a job she had been doing since the first day.

This group of individuals often had to literally make something out of nothing. The shuttle recovery operation's rapid growth and progress not only outpaced the supplies, but the needs also developed before the necessary funds were available. The federal government was footing the bill and the vast majority of the supplies coming in from private sources were being offered at cut rates, but the operation still needed finances of some sort. The obvious answer to this problem was credit. Almost all of the initial supplies that came out of the Logistics Section were purchased on credit. Permission was also obtained from Jasper County Sheriff Billy Rowels (who was currently over the operation's Water Search Branch) to charge items purchased in Jasper to the Jasper County Sheriff's Department.

When the National Guard began arriving in the area, they also required the services of the Logistics Section. However, the military proved to be more of an asset than a liability. A handful of guardsmen were assigned to assist Mark in obtaining and storing supplies. These soldiers were sent on many errands that simply couldn't have been handled by the understaffed Logistics Section. At one point the soldiers were sent to Buna to pick up a copier that had been donated by the Buna School District and they made several trips to Beaumont for supplies. In another instance, a group of soldiers were sent to Louisiana to shop for supplies at the Wal-Mart in Many.

Of course, the National Guardsmen weren't the only people running back and forth with supplies. Mark had temporarily moved his residence from Jasper to the Super 8 Motel on Toledo Bend Reservoir; however, he was still required to make several trips outside of the county. On one particular trip back to Hemphill from a FEMA briefing, he stopped off at Wal-Mart in Nacogdoches to pick up some batteries they had donated to the effort. The donation turned out to be larger than Mark had anticipated, and by the time he finished loading his trunk with boxes, the nose of his patrol car stuck high in the air and his back bumper was almost touching the ground. This wouldn't be the only such heavy-laden trip Mark would make.

Mark was the Chief of the Logistics Section on into the second week when the Forest Service began to slowly take over all aspects of the operation. However, the new leadership recognized his skills and retained him in the role of an advisor/assistant to the Logistics Section on into the third week.

* * *

When a high tech search that included U2 spy planes, satellite photos, and sonar listening devices, began to develop in an area that still had party line telephone service in some areas and had only given up the idea of outhouses a few decades ago, it's safe to say there was a bit of a technological gap. In the early

90s, while the Internet was booming around the world, we didn't have access here in Sabine County, unless you wanted to pay long distance charges while you were logged on, that is.

Albeit a fairly new service, we did have internet access when the shuttle crashed in 2003. In the mid-90s Jasnet out of Jasper had established the county's first local connection to the World Wide Web, and not long afterwards, locally owned Sabinenet came into existence.

As luck would have it, Sabinenet's offices were next door to the fire hall, so it was easy to run wire back and forth from the numerous computers springing up in the Incident Command Center to Sabinenet's main computer. Butch and Jaleen Andrews, who had purchased Sabinenet the year before the accident, gave free access to their computers to all organizations.

Also, Butch and Jaleen's son, Greg, was a Navy SEAL, and with the crisis in Afghanistan still simmering and the war with Iraq right around the corner, they fully understood how important it was for those who are away to remain in touch with those back at home. Throughout the recovery operation, they allowed any searchers who were away from home to send emails from their office free of charge.

Butch even took care of running the wires from his business to the Command Post. Once, while running one strand of wire over the heads of two NASA representatives at a desk, the wire slipped from the nails in the wall, knocking several sticky notes off of a map at their work station (no doubt Mark Allen would receive an order for thumbtacks from this station). The men at the desk looked up, affixing Butch with a questioning glare.

Butch said, "Look, I've got to do this. But if I'm going to do it, I'm going to do it right."

He returned to his office and got all the supplies he needed. Then he carefully ran the wire over the desks and across the fire hall's back office. When he was finished, one of the two NASA reps inspected his work and gave him a smile and a thumbs up.

Butch returned the gesture, and then got back to work running another line.

Logistics and communications in Sabine County would remain primary concerns throughout the operation. However, the hard work of skilled and determined individuals prevented this weak link from hindering the operation in the least. Columbia could hardly have come down in an area with worse terrain and fewer available resources. Luckily, she found a place with people who more than made up for this disadvantage.

12
Medical Response

D AVID WHITMIRE PULLED the ambulance into the parking lot across from the Hemphill Fire Hall. He and his partner, Don Rodriguez, climbed out of the cab and made their way across the street to the Command Center. David, a paramedic, and Don, an emergency medical technician, made up Med-10, one of Sabine County's two full time ambulance units. They were employees of Eastex, an ambulance service that operated in several counties in East Texas, including Sabine County.

David and Don were working a weekday-on, weekend-off schedule, and they had been off the day the shuttle crashed. However, like so many others in the area, they had been involved in the opening stages of the operation as volunteers. Both had helped their hometown as a volunteer those first two days— David assisting in Hemphill, Don in San Augustine.

Upon returning to work that Monday morning, Med-10 was assigned to the Incident Command Post. While all of the local paramedics were certainly familiar with the area, David was the only one born and raised in Sabine County. Normally basic knowledge of the roads and good dispatching was sufficient to keep the paramedics headed in the right direction. However, since the ambulance at the Command Center would be supporting the searchers in the woods, there was a good chance that the ambulance would be sent down trails and old logging roads if an emergency came up. It was decided that David's familiarity with the area could come in handy.

At first, Med-10 was worked into the organization at the Incident Command Post more as a readily available asset than an actual link or branch of the loose command structure. Stanley Christopher, the Police Chief of Jasper, was serving in the role of Safety Officer for the operation. He saw that all the local medical facilities and their assets were readily available. However, since the shuttle incident wasn't actually a medical disaster, there wasn't an actual Medical Division at the Command Post.

Since so much of Sabine County's resources were being utilized, Stanley needed someone who knew the area and who knew the people. As it turned out, he found just such a person in Hemphill's hardworking city manager, Don Iles. Iles was at the Command Post serving as the liaison for the city of Hemphill, and, since the operation headquarters was situated inside the city's fire hall, he had become one of the most active of the local volunteers. As a result, not only did he know the local contacts, but he knew the newcomers working at the command center and they knew him.

Almost as soon as they arrived that first morning, an unofficial link was established between Med-10 and Don Iles. If David had any questions or needed anything, he would ask Don Iles and he would carry the information on to Stanley or whoever the proper authority might be. Likewise, Stanley and the other leaders at the Command Post knew that he would keep the wires from getting crossed in their communications with the ambulance crew.

* * *

As it turned out, Med-10 was called into action early on their first morning at the Command Post. One of the searchers had fallen earlier in the morning and hurt her leg. Thinking she had only lightly sprained her ankle, the lady had decided to continue her search efforts. As she walked through the woods, her ankle continued to trouble her, but she managed to keep going until she fell a second time. This time the pain was excruciating, shooting all the way from her foot to her hip. The initial assessment at the site was that this poor woman might have a broken hip.

The call came over the radio that there was a person injured on one of the search teams. After receiving directions as to where the group had entered the woods, David and Don Rodriguez headed off. The plan was for the ambulance to drive about five miles outside the city limits and park near the buses. The ambulance crew would then walk on foot to the site, following a helicopter that was hovering over the scene.

Not long after Med-10 left the ICP, a third local "Don" came into the picture. Don Eddings, the U. S. Forestry official who was in charge of the helicopter search, was in the air at the time. Don knew the area well, and when he overheard the directions that the ambulance crew was given, he radioed Med-10 and gave the crew directions to another location that would get the ambulance much closer to the injured searcher.

Instead of taking Highway 87 South as previously ordered, David followed Don Eddings' directions down Springhill Road. Just outside the city limits, David turned down a dirt road and continued into a pasture. Once in the pasture, they turned behind a barn, where Don Eddings had said someone would be waiting to take them in.

Since the four-wheelers had proved so useful in reaching the crewmember site on Sunday, the leaders of the search teams had decided to separate a volunteer who was equipped with a four-wheeler from the walking teams for just such an emergency. They used Jason Pearson in this role today.

David parked the ambulance behind the barn and began loading all the necessary medical equipment on the back of Jason's four-wheeler. Once the backboard was secured in place, Don Rodriguez climbed on the back of the four-wheeler.

Jason and Don Rodriguez went on ahead while David brought up the rear on foot. In order to make the ride back as smooth as possible, David cleared the path as he walked, picking up any fallen branches that were in the path. There wasn't much of a path to and from the site, so the way back had been marked by tying flags to trees. Luckily, the underbrush in this area was relatively light. As it turned out, Don Eddings had cut the distance to the site in half with his directions; however, it was still a good mile down an old foot trail to the site. By the time the four-wheeler got so far ahead that David lost sight, he was beginning to feel he had been given the short end of the stick.

* * *

When Don Rodriguez and Jason arrived at the site, they found a group of Forest Service officials and members of the search team attempting to make the lady comfortable. Don unloaded the backboard and the equipment needed to secure the patient. With the help of several of the members of the team, Don placed the lady's leg in a splint from the hip down. They then placed her neck in a C collar, her head on a headrest, and carefully strapped her down on the backboard. As they carefully placed the backboard across the back of the four-wheeler, one of the members of the lady's search team commented, "We could tip her over and she wouldn't fall off."

David arrived just as they were getting ready to start back. He positioned two members of the search team in front of the four-wheeler to pick up any limbs he might have missed. Two more members of the team walked on either side of the four-wheeler, holding the backboard in place and David and Don brought up the rear.

Driving slowly down the newly prepared path, the ride back was a smooth one for their patient. The only real obstacle they encountered was a shallow creek. The cot was carefully removed from the four-wheeler and hefted across the creek by hand. They reloaded on the other side and slowly continued on their way.

Once they reached the barn, the patient was carefully loaded into the ambulance. She was then rushed to Sabine County Hospital where it was determined that her hip wasn't broken, but she did have a severely sprained ankle.

As soon as Med-10 had finished their run they returned to

the Command Post and went back on call, ready for any other emergency that might come up.

* * *

Throughout the following two weeks Med-10 remained stationed at the ICP. During this time, Don Iles continued to handle the radio and telephone contacts for the ambulance crew, as well all the verbal links with the various organizations involved.

On February 5, Stanley Christopher was reassigned to help the Texas Department of Criminal Justice, who were bringing in mounted officers to assist in the search. Brad Moore of the Texas Forest Service was now the new Safety Officer. For the most part, this transition worked without a hitch. A minor misunderstanding took place on Brad's first day when Med-10 responded to a 911 call in the Hemphill area. Some of the federal officials were unaware that the ambulance would still be responding to 911 calls, and, when they noticed the ambulance's absence, they wanted to know where the ambulance had gone. The dispatchers received an agitated phone call from the Command Post and the agitation was passed through the radio from the dispatcher to Med-10. However, the ambulance couldn't very well turn around on an emergency run. After this brief moment of confusion, Don Iles remedied the situation at the ICP, explaining that the ambulances were still needed by the local populace as well as the search operation.

Brad proved very understanding. He agreed to work out an arrangement where both the operation and the people of the county could benefit from the medical resources. That night he saw that the tasks of the ambulance crews were carefully ironed out. The next morning's Incident Action Plan identified each ambulance and stated its role in the operation. Med-10 would remain at the ICP, and respond to 911 calls in the Hemphill area. Med-4 would operate out of the Volunteer Staging Area, but spend most of its time in the Pineland area to answer 911 calls in that part of the county. The other two ambulances that had recently been brought in from outside the county would follow the two main search teams out and operate from their drop off point. These ambulances would be solely responsible for their teams and were not expected to answer 911 calls.

Around the middle of the second week the search began making its full transition to a federal operation. The medical services continued without skipping a beat.

* * *

During the first two weeks of the operation, the ambulance crews answered numerous calls. None of these calls proved as serious as that first call, but there were certainly enough twisted ankles to go around once the ground became wet. They also saw quite a few "snake bites," although the vast majority of these turned out to be a combination of thorn pricks and imaginative panic.

As the operation continued to grow, more ambulance teams came in from throughout the state. Most of these operated out of the Volunteer Staging Area. Also, many of the federal organizations and the Native American search teams that came to the area brought their own paramedics.

When the ICP at the fire hall closed down at the end of the second week, the local EMS crews were for the most part freed to return to normal duty. However, when the ICP moved to the VFW hall and Youth Arena rodeo grounds at the beginning of the third week, EMS operations continued much in the same manner, and they would still occasionally be called on to answer calls for the duration of the operation.

13
Lending a Hand

WHEN THE STUDENTS of Hemphill High School returned to class on Monday morning on the third day of the operation, the halls buzzed with questions and stories concerning the disaster. Quite a few students had to see themselves off to school that morning, since their parents had volunteered to search the woods and had already left home before the school bus arrived. Other students had helped their parents prepare food to take to the VFW hall over the weekend. Like the rest of the community, these kids wanted to be part of this national tragedy—they wanted to help.

Principal Steve Mills and counselor Marc Griffin had already realized how important it was to involve the students in what was going on. Not only were they a ready source of eager help, but such involvement would have other, longer reaching effects on the students. This would be an experience that would stay with them for a lifetime, and they would learn the value of volunteerism along the way.

There was, however, still a question of how the students could help. This was answered Monday afternoon when Belinda Gay called from the VFW hall. This was one of the hundreds of calls Belinda made that day to ask for food donations. She asked if some of the teachers might come up with some desserts and bring them to the VFW hall on Tuesday. She also asked if it was possible for a group of students to be sent out that morning to help clean up after the volunteers left for the woods.

Worried that too many students at one time might become

Finding Heroes
101

too disorganized, Steve and Marc decided to limit the number of students who could go to the VFW hall the next morning. Vermykia Proctor was put in charge of creating a signup sheet and limiting the number of volunteers. The students filled this sheet almost as soon as it appeared in the high school's front office. Other sheets were placed in the office for the rest of the week, and they, too, were soon filled. In fact, Vermykia had to go back and weed out the students who had signed up for multiple days so that everyone who was interested could be involved.

Since this school outing had come on such short notice, it was impossible to go by the standard school procedure. Instead of sending a note home for the parents to sign, the high school attempted to call the parent of every student who had signed up in order to obtain permission for their child to go to the VFW hall. However, with so many of the local population out lending a hand, quite a few of the parents weren't home. Luckily, since it was a local trip which was going to be directly supervised by the high school principal, it was decided that parental consent was optional.

* * *

Tuesday morning, after first and second period classes, Steve loaded about a dozen teenagers into the school's van and drove them out to the VFW hall. They arrived just after the buses had left carrying the volunteers out to search the woods.

The students were put to work almost as soon as they got out of the van. One group cleaned the tables, another group swept the floor, and another group helped straighten the kitchen. This bit of help was a godsend for the weary cooks who had been working steadily since four o'clock that morning. It allowed them to take a break and have coffee and breakfast themselves.

Once the kitchen and the hall were clean, the students helped the cooks prepare the sack lunches that the Red Cross would be taking out into the field for the searchers' break. Each of these bags contained two sandwiches—one meat and cheese and one peanut butter and jelly. It also contained a fruit—either an apple, an orange, or a banana—and two snacks—a granola bar and a candy bar. Once they were prepared and sacked, the sandwiches were placed in boxes for transportation to the day's midway point.

After the sack lunches were on their way to the searchers, the students were loaded up and taken back to the school. Over the next two weeks, Hemphill and West Sabine High Schools would alternate sending volunteers to the VFW hall. Over the weekend various church youth groups would take up where the schools had left off, sending their own groups to lend a hand.

* * *

The Hemphill school district's role in the recovery operation didn't end with their employees' food donations and their students' trips to the VFW hall. Near the middle of the first week, the National Guard began arriving to assist in the search. The school offered the use of their gym to house the soldiers. The Guard refused the offer to quarter the troops on campus, but they were interested in using the gym's showers.

The National Guard's first night in Hemphill was a miserable one. With only a handful of port-o-potties and no shower stalls, they pitched tents on the sandy ground at the rodeo arena. They had to drive into town to take their showers at the high school, and once they were there, the old gym's water heater would only support the first few who hit the showers. After that, it was a miserable, icy shower. The next day the guardsmen changed their mind. They moved into the school's old gym, and their Hummers and heavy-duty trucks took over the students' parking lot.

Initially there was some concern about the possibility of a volatile combination of teenagers and soldiers. However, it soon became clear there would be no problem whatsoever. For one thing, the guardsmen were gone most of the day, and when they were there, they were exceedingly polite and respectful. When the soldiers were available, they were more than willing to take the students out and show them their vehicles and equipment. Despite the strange circumstances of their arrival, the soldiers didn't serve as the least bit of a distraction. In fact, the only noticeable change in the student body was in fashion. Many of the students wore their hunting gear to school as camouflage suddenly came in style.

The National Guard found the facilities at the high school a huge improvement over their one night stay at the rodeo arena. The heater and solid roof over their heads was a vast improvement over their military issue tents.

Also, now that the community was fully aware of their arrival, on their second day in Hemphill they became the sudden target of Sabine County's hospitality. People brought home-cooked snacks, and even a television and a VCR. The greatest gift, however, came from the school district—later in the week the gym's old hot water heater was replaced by a brand new, much larger one. It's odd how some of the luxuries we take for granted come to the forefront once we are without them—the warm showers were a huge hit with the soldiers.

* * *

The high school also provided entertainment for the soldiers in the form of our district basketball games. On the first Tuesday night, the soldiers packed into our new gym to watch our Hemphill Hornets trounce the Timpson Bears. We had a good team that year; we'd only lost one district game. However, that one game was a loss to the Woden Eagles, whom we were to play again that Friday.

When Friday came, camouflage fatigues filled the home side of the new gym, but from the first tip-off, Woden's excellent team dominated the first half, jumping out to a lead of around twenty points. When the second half started, the soldiers started cheering and taking up chants, encouraging our team. Apparently the hospitality had given them a feeling of home that was now paying dividends. With the guardsmen encouraging them on, our boys managed to whittle away at the Eagles lead and pull within a couple of baskets before losing the game in the last few seconds.

On the second Tuesday of the operation we were scheduled to play our arch-rivals, the San Augustine Wolves. Seeing the fun that the guardsmen had at the game and the positive effect on our players, efforts were made to secure a bus to take them to the game. However, considering how the guard filled our gym, there was no way San Augustine's smaller gym could hold both sets of fans, our guardsmen, and the guardsmen who were in San Augustine for the search.

In the short period that the National Guard was in Sabine County, they truly became a part of our community, and, judging by the number of them who said they were going to move here some day, we found a place in their hearts as well.

14

Bronson's Dogs

S AN EMPLOYEE of the Texas Parks and Wildlife, Lin Marcantel of Bronson was a very busy man during the first few days of the operation. On Monday morning he drove over to the Bannister Wildlife Refuge near the border of Sabine and San Augustine Counties. He spent the better part of the day searching through the refuge on a four-wheeler but found nothing of great significance.

On his way back home that afternoon, Lin stopped by Lance and Charles Connor's house in Bronson. They stood in the front yard for several minutes, discussing the shuttle disaster and the ongoing recovery operation.

During their conversation, Charles mentioned that he had heard something crash in the woods behind the house and that they had just gotten around to calling the sheriff's department, so Lin was aware that a group was on their way from Hemphill to investigate their call. However, Lin was fully unprepared for the armada of cars that suddenly descended on the place. Several unmarked cars carrying one of the FBI recovery teams suddenly rounded the corner and pulled in at the Connors's.

A big-boned blonde lady in an FBI windbreaker climbed out of one of the cars and hurried over toward the group. She immediately approached Lin and began asking questions and taking notes on a notepad clamped onto a clipboard. She glanced at the patch on Lin's shoulder and asked who he was and what organization he was with.

"Lin Marcantel, with the Texas Parks and Wildlife."

"Have you investigated their report?"

"No, I haven't."

"Why did you call us out here?"

"I didn't call you. I just happened to stop by right before you showed up."

The agent continued directing her questions toward Lin while Lance and Charles looked on in silence. Finally, Lin told the lady, "Look, you need to be talking to them. They heard the noise, and they called you out here."

The agent turned and directed a few questions toward Lance and Charles, but after only a few minutes she once again turned her attention back to Lin. When a second attempt to convince the lady that she was questioning the wrong person fell on deaf ears, he walked away from the group, hoping his absence would solve the problem.

Much to his surprise, when he turned around, he found the agent had followed him. It was as if this woman was completely uncomfortable talking with common people and had to locate someone in a uniform to field her questions. Seeing that his presence was strangely distracting, Lin was left with no choice but to leave the Connors' place completely.

When he pulled into his own drive, he half expected to see that strange FBI agent pull in the drive behind him. She didn't arrive that night, but he hadn't heard the last of her.

* * *

The next day Lin was planning to spend the day riding with Chad Gartman, a Game Warden out of Newton. They were going to drive along the various backroads and trails in and near the shuttle's flight corridor. However, before Lin could get out the door, his wife, Amy called. Amy, who worked at the sheriff's office as a dispatcher, said that the sheriff wanted Lin to get a map of Bronson and go to the Bronson fire hall. Chief Deputy Chad Murray would meet him there.

After Lin found a good map of Bronson, he and Chad

Gartman left for the fire hall. When they pulled into the drive, Chad Murray was waiting for them in his patrol car.

"Do you know anything about any unmarked graves around here?" Chad asked.

"This is Bronson, Texas," Lin replied with a smile. "Just about everybody has an unmarked grave or two in their backyard."

"I want your opinion on something," Chad said, turning to lead the way around the fire hall.

Behind the fire hall, Chad showed Lin a rough circular hole in the ground, about two feet in diameter and about a foot and a half deep. A few bones, partially covered by dirt, were apparent in the bottom of the shallow grave. The hole was wide open, and there wasn't any fresh dirt, so it appeared as if someone hadn't even bothered to properly cover it.

Chad told Lin that an FBI agent had discovered these bones and decided that she had discovered an unsolved murder in Bronson. She had called the sheriff's department to set up an investigation, but Sheriff Maddox had already dealt with her the day before. He figured she didn't know what she was talking about—it was only her second day in East Texas, but this agent from the big city had already managed to agitate just about everyone she had dealt with. Tom sent Chad out to investigate the so-called mystery grave, and, once he had arrived, Chad had called for Lin in order to get a second opinion.

Lin stooped down and peered into the grave. The bones were old, but there was still a lot of hide in the grave as well— enough to give Lin a perfect idea as to what he was looking at.

"Well, it's one of two things," Lin said. "It's either a dog's grave, or someone has buried Tommy Welch back here." (Tommy Welch was a particularly hairy resident of Bronson.)

Chad agreed, but since the FBI was running the show, he decided to let Terry Lane have a look at the grave before they officially closed the little pseudo investigation.

* * *

When Terry arrived, he was led up to the hole. He didn't even have to stoop down to see the obvious. "Yeah, it's a dog."

Of course, Terry had never met Tommy Welch.

* * *

The FBI agent's attempt to clean up this one horse town didn't stop with one embarrassing episode behind the fire hall. Apparently she had come to Texas to make a name for herself, because she was bound and determined to find an unsolved mystery in the piney woods.

At approximately the same time Terry, Lin, and both Chads were investigating her first unsolved mystery, she was conjuring up an even greater monstrosity only a couple blocks away at the First Baptist Church of Bronson. This time she had discovered a mass burial site behind the church. Bones littered the grounds behind the building, protruding from graves that were often nothing more than a thin layer of dirt. To this city-bred agent, the scene must have looked like something straight out of H. P. Lovecraft's worst nightmares—perhaps she had uncovered some sort of sick, twisted religious cult. Once again, the agent called the sheriff's office. This time she wanted an FBI forensics team and a Texas Ranger sent out to the scene, pronto. Once again, Chad Murray pulled the duty of chasing this lady's wild geese.

As it turned out, this time her discovery was even more laughable that the one behind the fire hall, and, once again, dogs were involved. Apparently someone living near the church was an avid hunter, because some neighborhood dogs had made off with several deer bones and buried them behind the church.

15

The Fourth Day's Recoveries

THE NEXT MORNING I discovered that my suit situation was critical. I didn't have a single suit hanging in my closet. Every suit I owned was either at the cleaners or covered with mud. I piled all my suits into the passenger's seat of my car, and hurried to the cleaners, where I dropped off and picked up my laundry. I found that I only had one suit ready to be picked up. However, we didn't have any bodies in the funeral home, so I could get by with blue jeans and a collared shirt. I returned home and put my suit in the closet.

Dad wasn't there when I arrived at the Funeral Home, so I gave him a call. We talked for a while and he mentioned that he was tired and trying to get some rest this morning. Not only had he been working later than myself due to the daily trips to Lufkin, but he had also been busy taking care of his sick mother for several weeks before the shuttle accident. I suggested he take the day off, but he said he only needed a little nap. He would be coming in around noon.

Noon came and went quietly without word from either the command center or my father. We had been called in at three o'clock yesterday and the day before, and as the afternoon wore on without any sign of my father, I began to realize I was probably going to be on my own today. This was fine with me. The first day jitters were far behind me, and I felt I could handle any situation that came up. I was actually a little disappointed when Dad pulled into the driveway right at three o'clock.

When I met him at the back door, he immediately asked why

I wasn't in a suit. I explained my situation, but he wasn't satisfied. I attempted to lighten the mood by pulling his leg. I told him it was easy for him to wear a suit every day since he owned around two dozen; myself, I only owned four—I suggested a raise. Apparently, Dad wasn't in good spirits today, because the joke fell flat and almost caused an argument. I knew he was tired and irritable, so I quickly agreed to run home and change.

However, I didn't make it out the door before the command center called. Another body had been found. Instead of sending us to the command center, they gave us directions over the phone in order to save time. We were to leave Hemphill on Highway 83, the site wasn't far outside of the city limits. We would see the cars.

We climbed in the Excursion and immediately got underway, my father grumbling about my attire the entire way.

About three miles outside city limits we came up on a row of unmarked cars lining the road. We noticed several people in FBI shirts in the area, but I didn't recognize any of them. Apparently, this was a *third* recovery team.

Thankfully, my father's grumbling switched from myself to the fact that the FBI had so many teams working the area. There was no way to tell if we needed to pull into the pasture or stay on the road, so Dad pulled up to the first agent he saw and rolled down the window on my side. "Where do you want us?" he asked.

The agent either didn't hear him, or wasn't sure what to say, because he just stood there. When Dad repeated the question, the agent pointed to a lady getting out of a car up from us and said she was in charge of the recovery team.

Dad drove on and pulled up beside the agent in charge of the team. "Where do you want us?" he asked again.

She affixed him with a questioning look. "Who are you?"

"Squeaky Starr."

"What agency are you with?"

"We're with the funeral home. We've been helping with the recovery and transportation of the remains."

"*We* do the recovery," she said in an abrupt I'm-the-one-in-charge-here tone that I knew wouldn't set well with my already irritable father. "I'll let you know when I need you for transportation."

"Do you want us to go back?" Dad snapped. His temper was building and his patience was wearing thin.

As for myself, caught in between the two as I was, I began slowly sinking in my seat.

Now the lady suddenly didn't seem so sure of herself. Perhaps she realized that if she hadn't been the one to call us out, someone else had to have made the call. "Yeah, I'll call when . . ."

Without letting her finish, Dad rolled up the window, turned the Excursion around, and started back to town. He picked up the mike on our police radio. "299 to Hemphill."

"Go ahead 299."

"We're 10-22." That's ten code for aborting a call.

* * *

When we returned to town, Dad went to the law enforcement center instead of the command center. He told me he was going to run in and let them know why he had left the scene, and then return to the funeral home.

I didn't stick around to see what was said. I realized my father was tired, stressed, and irritable. My lack of a suit may or may not have been part of the problem, but I wasn't going to take any chances. While he went inside, I walked to the road and thumbed a ride to the funeral home where I could pick up my car and rush home. Once home, I got out of my jeans and into a suit.

Only a few minutes after I had left, my little black Mustang slid into the parking lot in front of the law enforcement center. Despite my haste, I missed my father. He had already been recalled to the scene. However, I was only a minute or so behind him. I pulled out of the drive and headed toward the site.

I pulled up to the scene just as Dad was getting out of the Excursion. He glanced at me as I got out of my car, noticed the suit, but didn't say a word.

None of the agents were at their cars. They had joined Terry and the astronaut at the site, which was actually several hundred yards into the woods.

No sooner had I joined my father at the Excursion than we saw the recovery team coming out of the woods at the far back of the pasture. Seconds later, Terry appeared out of the woods behind them. When he saw me and my father standing by the road waiting on them, he literally broke into a run in order to beat the recovery team to us and avoid a possible second confrontation.

When he reached us, he apologized for the agent's behavior. Dad once again mentioned that everything would go a lot smoother if there was only one recovery team to work with.

"As soon as we break a team in, they send someone new," Dad said with a smile. This was the first bit of humor I'd heard from him today.

Terry laughed and agreed that they were a little overloaded with personnel.

Dad and Terry then discussed what had taken place when we arrived the first time. Terry explained that the agent hadn't been briefed on our involvement in the recovery, and that she was just going "by the books." However, he agreed that a little common courtesy and common sense on her part could have solved the issue before it became a problem.

By now the recovery team was coming out of the pasture. Terry called them over and introduced us. With the usual Terry Lane tact, he told them that we had been with the operation since day one and, while we weren't part of any agency, we were part of this recovery operation. The agent over the recovery team apologized. Even though the misunderstanding wasn't their fault, the other agents on her team also apologized as they took turns shaking our hands

When the recovery team started back to their cars, Terry and a few of the agents who were at the scene with him but not part of that particular team stayed and spoke with my father. These were some of the agents who had been here since the first day. Several of those who stayed behind seemed highly agitated at the recovery team leader's behavior. I would later find out that this hadn't been this agent's first blunder in Sabine County. She was the same agent who had been so convinced that our local dogs were actually rampant murderers. The next day would prove to be another story. Much to our surprise the over-eager agent had undergone an overnight transformation. Even my father, who is certainly the type to hold grudges, admitted that she had actually calmed down to the point of being easy to work with. It's a shame she had already stepped on so many toes.

I was so caught up in the conversation with the agents that it was some time before I noticed that they had returned from the site without a body bag. I asked Terry about the body, and he told me that they found a four-wheeler trail and a small group had decided to take the body out by this longer, but less dense path.

The next portion of this recovery was something I was growing quite accustomed to—waiting. We stood around the vehicles for about thirty minutes before Terry received a call on his cell phone. Apparently, the four-wheeler trail had proved considerably longer than they had believed. The group carrying the body had finally reached the edge of the woods, but they were almost a mile farther down the road.

Everyone loaded into a vehicle. In order to cut down on a little of the parking clutter, I left my Mustang and climbed in the Excursion with Dad.

Not far down the road, we were flagged down by a lone agent. The cars ahead and behind us pulled off the shoulder of the road and we were directed to back down a dirt road that was blocked from the highway by a locked iron gate.

The group appeared out of the edge of the woods and started toward the gate. Texas Ranger Danny Young and Fred Raney were among the small group carrying the body bag, as was a small short-haired lady in a blue astronaut's jumpsuit. I helped the group over the gate, and loaded the body bag into the back of the Excursion.

While my father spoke with Terry, I stayed with Fred, Danny and the astronaut near the back of the Excursion. The lady in the blue jumpsuit was astronaut Nancy Currie, and she proved to be quite an interesting person. Nancy had served as mission specialist on four shuttle missions, including STS-109, Columbia's previous mission. She was very soft-spoken and down to earth, certainly not what you would expect from someone who had orbited the planet 648 times.

When Dad joined us, he asked Nancy about Mark Kelley. On Saturday morning, Mark had been thrown into an operation to recover seven friends and coworkers with only a few hours notice. While he hadn't faltered in the least while undertaking this painful task, it was apparent that he needed a break. Nancy replied that Mark had gone home for some much needed rest. She also mentioned that there were several others at NASA who were also having trouble dealing with the current tragedy. This was just like a sudden, tragic death in a close-knit family.

When we broke up our conversation, Nancy replaced me in the Excursion. They had decided to make this run to Lufkin through Pineland. There were enough FBI agents with us to provide a suitable escort.

Once the crewmember was on its way to Lufkin, Terry gave me a lift back to my car. Despite the misunderstanding between my father and the leader of the recovery team, today's operation had gone quite smoothly. In fact, for the first time in four days, I pulled into the driveway at my house well before sunset. Little did I know I would be called back to the command center within the hour.

* * *

My wife was at a basketball game, so I had the house to myself. I poured a glass of lemonade, sat down in my recliner, and turned on the news for the first time in four days. Aside from taking off my jacket at the door and loosening my tie, I didn't even bother to get out of my suit.

I watched the news for all of five minutes before I realized that the last thing I wanted to do was to watch the news reports on the recovery operation. I needed to take a break and put all of this behind me for a couple of hours.

I changed the channel to the Cartoon Network. One of those Robot Kung Fu cartoons was on, but as much as I can't stand Japanimation, this would have to do. Sure enough, it did the trick. A few laser-blasted battle-bots later, I nodded off in my chair.

Although I was probably out for the better part of a half an hour, the phone seemed to ring as soon as my head slumped onto my chest. The portable phone was in the kitchen. In my haste to get into relax mode, I had forgotten to take the phone with me to the living room. At first I was in no hurry to get to the phone. I knew I was on call to go out if they found another site, but I doubted they would have found something this late in the day. It was probably just another reporter.

When I reached the phone on the umpteenth ring and saw the Sheriff's Department number on my caller I.D., I almost flipped out.

I snatched the portable phone out of its cradle. "Hello?"

"Byron, this is the Sheriff's Office," the dispatcher said. "They've got something else they want you to take to Lufkin."

"Do I need to run by the Command Post for directions?"

"No, they've already brought it in. They want you to come to the Sheriff's Office and back up to the sally port."

"Okay. I'm on my way."

* * *

On my way to the funeral home to pick up the hearse, I realized one minor detail I had overlooked. I didn't know how to get to Dr. Bruce's. Our county had been using Dr. Bruce as their pathologist for decades. However, since I graduated mortuary school, he had always sent a car to pick up and return the bodies to our funeral home. As a result, I had never actually taken a body to his lab.

I knew someone at the sheriff's office probably knew how to get there, but I didn't want to take any chances. When I got to the funeral home I went into the office and rifled through Virginia's rolodex until I found Dr. Bruce's card. However, when I dialed the number, I didn't get an answer. His home phone number was on the back of the card, so I tried it. Still no answer. Frustrated, I tossed the card onto the desk, grabbed the keys to the hearse and darted out the back door.

* * *

When I arrived at the Sheriff's Office, an agent was in the parking lot waiting for me. He told me they found a crew-related item when the search groups were coming in that afternoon. Another cooler was waiting for me inside the sally port.

I backed into the open gate and another agent placed the cooler in the back of the hearse while the first went to find an escort. I saw Shane approaching from the direction of the command center and hurried to meet him.

"We've got one little problem," I said.

"What's that?"

"I've never been to Dr. Bruce's," I replied.

He told me not to worry about it. He would find someone to lead me who had already made the trip.

While Shane tried to locate someone, I went inside the Sheriff's Office to use the phone. There was no doubt in my mind that Shane would come through, but I had rather find the directions on my own if at all possible. I went into the booking room to use the phone. I tried calling my father's cell phone, but he didn't answer—he seldom turned the thing on anyway. I was about to call Debi to see if she could give me some quick directions when the dispatcher across the hall told me Shane was outside looking for me. That was quick!

Shane quickly introduced me to the agent in charge of the evidence, and my ride-along astronaut. As it turned out, the astronaut had been to the lab the day before, and he would serve as my guide.

With all the details ironed out, we all climbed in our vehicles and headed to Lufkin. Unlike my father's four prior trips to Lufkin, this one was done with little fanfare. The hearse was in the lead, followed by the evidence agent, who also served as my official escort.

The funny thing about this trip was I never managed to get the astronaut's name. When Shane introduced us, I was still so worked up about not knowing how to get to Dr. Bruce's office that the man's name went in one ear and out the other. Like all the other astronauts I had met thus far, this guy was polite and friendly. This one was also full of questions. It took an hour to get to Lufkin, and for the entire trip he asked question after question about my profession and my hometown. It was truly amazing that a person with so much education, experience and adventure in their background could be interested in my simple life. His curiosity was charming, almost like that of a child, and refreshing in a way. It dawned on me that one doesn't get to where this man was in life without having a serious hunger for knowledge.

When we reached Lufkin, we pulled around to the back of the small building near Woodland Heights Medical Center. A Federal Marshal directed me to back up to the double doors.

I had already met one interesting character in the nameless astronaut, now I was about to meet another. I had overheard Terry and a few of the other agents telling my father about the forensics expert in charge at Lufkin. According to all accounts, she was good—damn good. And like all good forensics experts, she had a few little quirks. It has been my experience that a pathologist in his or her lab is like a captain on his ship. While they're usually a lot more upbeat than Hollywood likes to portray them, they still can be quite territorial about their labs. They don't care if you're the President or the Pope, they're in charge while you're on their turf. This lady added a little twist of humor to that professional territorialism—she liked to be called "Queen" while she was at work.

However, unlike my meeting with the astronaut, my meeting with Queen was brief and almost wordless. She ushered me into the lab, took the cooler, then ushered me out. The entire exchange consisted of "Thank you" and "You're welcome."

My new astronaut friend would be staying in Lufkin, so I started back to Hemphill alone. In contrast to the ride to Lufkin, the ride back was quiet and boring.

16
Trudging Through the Cold Rain

CHIP ROBBERSON WAS the Line Manager for Million Air, a Fixed Base Operator at Wiley Post Airport in Bethany, Oklahoma. He had been a licensed pilot for over twenty years, and on January 12, 2001, he married his wife Teresa in Million Air's hangar. At the beginning of the ceremony, Teresa taxied into the hangar in a Citation Jet. Chip had arranged for a helicopter to pick them up after the ceremony and take them to them to their honeymoon hotel, but the weather canceled the flight.

Aviation was Chip's life. He grew up watching the Mercury, Gemini, and Apollo flights and when the Space Shuttle Challenger exploded after liftoff back on January 28, 1986, he felt his heart sink. On February 1, 2003, that terrible feeling returned when he heard that Columbia had fallen apart upon reentry. He and his wife spent all day watching the news, and finally it was more than he could take. He asked his wife if she would be okay with him going down to East Texas and helping in the recovery operation. Teresa understood that this was very important to him and was supportive of his decision. He spoke to his employer, asking if he could use some of his vacation time on short notice. As with his wife, his request was met with understanding. Chip was given time off and even allowed to use a company car to make the trip.

Before he left, Chip didn't really talk much about his planned trip to East Texas. He felt an odd mixture of excitement and sadness over the coming trip. He was elated to be able to lend a hand and to help bring the remains of heroes and fellow aviators home to their loved ones, but there was no escaping the gloom of the recent tragedy.

Chip knew from watching the news that the shuttle's crewmembers were being found around Hemphill, in the Sabine County area. That was where Chip wanted to be. On Tuesday morning he called the Sabine County Sheriff's Department and asked how to go about volunteering for the recovery effort. The dispatcher told him that the town's VFW hall was the Volunteer Staging Area and gave him the number. Chip called the VFW hall. They told him that all help was greatly appreciated.

Just in case he had to sleep in his car, Chip picked a station wagon out of the company vehicles. He knew he wouldn't be able to make the long drive in time to take part in that day's search, but he would be there in plenty of time to help on the next day.

* * *

When Chip arrived at the VFW hall, the busloads of volunteers were beginning to return from the woods. Chip found a parking place as close to the VFW hall as possible and walked the rest of the way. The first person Chip met when he came through the door was Tony Alexander. A Navy veteran, Tony was not only a member of the local VFW, he was also the VFW District Commander; however, today he was here as a volunteer with the Six Mile Fire Department. Chip explained his reason for being here, and Tony asked if he would like to eat with their group.

Tony led Chip to the table and introduced him to the others. Chip was impressed with the group as soon as he met them. They were tired, worn, and hungry, but every person at that table was quick with a friendly greeting and a smile.

Once everyone had settled in and started eating, Tony began quizzing Chip. Throughout the operation, several volunteers had arrived who had no business in the woods. Tony respected their enthusiasm, but these out of shape individuals could prove a liability to the line. And physical fitness wasn't the only worry on Tony's mind. He looked Chip dead in the eye when he mentioned that this was where the astronauts were being found. Chip replied that this was why he had come here and that he was prepared for such a discovery, emotionally and otherwise—one of his past jobs had been working surgery in Oklahoma. Tony smiled and told Chip to be ready bright and early in the morning because he would be part of Group 3.

Chip was honored, and impressed.

* * *

When Bob Morgan awoke Wednesday morning, he found his flu was trying to stage a comeback. His wife was worried about his health. She wanted him to stay home, but he insisted that he needed to at least go in to see how everything was going before the searchers once again hit the woods. It was cold out and sleet was falling miserably from the dark sky that morning; this was going to be a grueling day on the line. Nevertheless, as soon as Bob convinced his wife he was only going to the volunteer staging area for the morning briefing, he slipped over to the Six Mile fire hall and replaced his ruined wildlands suit with a heavy jacket and gathered several other items he would need for walking the woods.

Although he was now fully prepared, Bob was still undecided as to whether or not he should walk the line today. There was little doubt that his health had taken a turn for the worse, but he desperately wanted to be a part of the operation. When Bob arrived at the VFW hall, Jason presented him with a walking stick. Jason had located the stick the night before while making a private search of the woods around his house. It appeared to be an old surveyor's stick. When Bob was presented with the stick, the gesture made up his mind for him. He was going out again.

Not long after breakfast, Bob called his wife to let her know he was going out. Apparently she already knew what was on his mind. He only managed to get out a couple of words before she shouted, "I knew it! I knew you were going out there!" and slammed the phone down onto the receiver.

* * *

Chip slept on a cot in the back of the VFW hall his first night in town. A rough bed in such a noisy place certainly didn't make for a good night's sleep, but at least when he awoke the next morning getting breakfast and coffee was only a matter of walking into the next room. He was filling his plate with eggs when the lady serving coffee asked where he was staying. He replied that he was staying in the back room of the VFW hall. Without giving it a second thought, the lady said, "I have an extra bedroom at my house, and you will stay with me tonight." Chip was shocked and amazed that someone would open their house to a complete stranger. The lady introduced herself as Pat Oden. She said that she would wash his clothes and make him supper as well. Chip said he didn't want to be a bother, but she insisted. She told him to call her when he got back from the search and she would give him directions to her house.

Chip was still recovering from this shock of kindness when he walked up to the table for a refill of coffee. A black lady behind the table asked where he was from, and he told her. When she heard how far he had traveled she replied, "Well, while you're here I'm your black mother. If you need anything, let me know."

Chip didn't know what to say. These two encounters had just reaffirmed the feeling that there was something special going on in Sabine County. He now knew beyond a shadow of a doubt that he had done the right thing in coming here.

* * *

When the veteran members of Group 3 started trickling into the VFW hall, they were every bit as impressed with Chip as he had been with them the day before. Despite Tony's line of questioning, most of the searchers expected the uninitiated city boy to show up in blue jeans, tee shirt and tennis shoes. However, he arrived wearing heavy woodlands clothes similar to theirs and carrying a machete. He was better prepared for his first day in the woods than many on the team had been on their first day.

Chip was a fresh face, and he was very upbeat and outgoing. Not only did his presence increase the line by one volunteer, but he proved to be a great morale boost. He would later comment how everyone else seemed upbeat and ready to go, but, in truth, many of the volunteers were getting tired. Like Bob, many of the searchers were nursing colds or fighting off the flu. Most of them weren't in the best of shape and these three hard days had pushed their bodies to the limit, not to mention the mental strain of the tragedy itself.

When they loaded into the bus, Chip noticed that just about everyone on board became quiet as they mentally prepared themselves for the task ahead. As for himself, Chip was once again feeling that odd mixture of excitement and sadness. He imagined that feeling was similar to what the others on the bus were experiencing.

As soon as they arrived at the drop off point, the team piled out of the buses. They were given another short briefing by one of the police officers who would be following along behind the lines. The officer gave everyone a brief reminder as to why they were here and what they were to look out for. He then went on to remind them about the wet slippery conditions and the other natural obstacles, such as the local wildlife, especially snakes and wild hogs. After their morning reminder, the team was stretched out along the line, with about ten feet between each searcher. Today a TV crew and a handful of photographers would be following along behind the line. They promised not to get in the way.

Everyone focused on the ground as they pushed through the cold mist. After an hour, the line reached a barbwire fence running alongside a dirt road. As Chip climbed over the top strand, a bright flash from a photographer's camera came from seemingly out of nowhere. It turned out the photographer was standing right next to him, but Chip had been so focused on watching the ground that he never realized there was anyone around other than his fellow volunteers.

As they pressed on, the team moved into heavier terrain. At times they could go no further than a few feet in five or ten minutes as the searchers had to hack away at the dense underbrush ahead. At times a volunteer would find himself severely tangled in the briars. The line would slow down and sometimes stop as the poor person tried to untangle himself. At one point Bob Morgan found himself in a tangle with a thorn buried deep in his lip. Todd Parish had to wade into a patch of briars to help Bob get untangled.

As they walked, Chip found out that the man walking to his right was also not from Sabine County. The man was David Brady, and he and Chip had a lot in common. They were both aviators, and had come to East Texas with a strong desire to lend a hand. David's involvement, however, was even more personal. He was a NASA employee who worked in Mission Control.

Chip and David talked back and forth as they waded through the brush, often playfully laughing at each other's misfortune. This laughter was stopped abruptly when David suddenly stopped and declared he had found something. Chip saw a white piece of bone in the brush ahead. He advanced slowly forward, his mind whirling with a mixture of emotions. However, when they cleared the brush from around the area, it proved to be an animal's skull. Chip's heart sank. His reason for being here was to bring Columbia's crewmembers back home and this had proved to be a false call.

At a little after noon, the searchers stopped for lunch. Being a pilot, Chip prided himself on always being able to tell which direction was north, south, east, and west. However, the East Texas woods had him completely lost; the tall pines hid all of the sky save a small patch directly overhead. Chip took a seat at the foot of a tall pine and ate one of the ready-to-eat meals. A cool breeze was blowing through the woods. It felt good.

The break only lasted twenty to thirty minutes. Group 3 was once again stretched out into a long line. Not long after their break, a searcher not far down the line from Chip stumbled on a moderate sized piece of debris, about six inches in diameter. Forest Service officials moved to the location, marked the area and got the GPS coordinates while the line continued pushing forward.

* * *

Near the center of Six Mile's portion of the line, Bob Morgan was finally beginning to play out. He had already been worn and weary when they stopped for lunch, but he had refused to call it quits. He continued pressing on through the afternoon, but he was now having to focus more on keeping his footing and less at watching the ground. Finally, when they were in the last half-mile of the day's search, he asked to be replaced on the line while he took a breather. After he caught his breath, Bob got back to his feet and fell in behind the line.

Despite all the hard work he put in, Bob felt a strange pang of guilt at having fallen out of line that day. Anyone could see that there was no need for this feeling; he had certainly put in his time and given his all. The fact that he could push himself this hard and still feel guilt over having not gone a few more feet shows how much the whole operation meant to Bob, and to us all. For thirteen days the recovery of Columbia and her crew became Sabine County's one and only purpose, and we certainly weren't going to fail for lack of trying.

* * *

The team continued until they reached an old logging road. This was their assigned drop-off point, and they had reached it just in time—darkness was falling fast. While they were waiting, the searchers of Group 3 found out that they had been the only search team to finish their designated area. This brought on a round of good-natured jabs at the other search teams. One of the members suggested a name for Team 3 and everyone agreed. And this is how Bobi Stiles' Group 3 came to be unofficially known as "The Hard Asses."

* * *

Pat Oden proved to be good for her word. Chip called as soon as he returned to the fire hall and she gave directions to her house out on the lake. She even drove out to the entrance of the subdivision to make sure he didn't get lost. One of the first things Chip did when he got to her house was take a much-needed shower. After he got out of the shower, Chip and Pat talked for a while. After almost nodding off on the couch in the middle of a conversation, Chip decided it was time to get some sleep. Pat said she would get him up in time for him to be out at the VFW hall the next morning.

Chip still found it hard to believe the warm welcome he was receiving. And Pat, for her part, was very impressed by Chip. She would later recall that he was the only man she'd ever met who actually cleaned up after himself in the bathroom.

17

A Privilege

WE HAD BEEN BLESSED with good weather over the first four days of the operation, but Wednesday saw a drop in the temperature and drizzling rain. The search continued, but there were rumors that it might be postponed until the rain let up.

When Dad came to work that morning, I asked to speak to him in his office. Once we were alone, I suggested he take a break. I could tell he was tired—before the shuttle incident even began he had already stretched himself thin by having to care for his sick mother; now he was exhausted. At first he claimed that he was fine, but I insisted that he needed the break and that I could handle anything that came up. I told him that if we ended up getting two calls at the same time he could run the second one. Dad finally agreed. He had a few phone calls to make, but as soon as he was finished, he said he would go home and get some rest.

While Dad was making his phone calls, I decided to drop by the ICP to let Shane and Terry know it was going to be me that would be on call. Before going to the command post, I stopped by the Sheriff's Office to let the dispatchers know that they needed to contact me rather than Dad if something came up. As it turned out, I didn't even have to go over to the ICP. When I stepped out of the sheriff's office, I found Terry in the parking lot. I told him that I would be first out today and Dad would be backing me up. That was fine with him; he said he would pass the word on to Shane.

Terry also mentioned that he had talked to Dad yesterday about our services. He said my father insisted that we were working for free, but Terry told me that the money was going to come out of FEMA, not NASA. He wanted me to tell Dad to be sure to send in a bill, because we deserved reimbursement for our work. I told him I would pass the message on.

* * *

While I was gone to town, Dad made a phone call to the Texas Funeral Service Commission. While we were currently working within a federal operation, the funeral industry normally answers to State law. We had been told not to file death certificates on the remains we were finding, but we needed official confirmation from the State to make sure we weren't violating any regulations. They told us that the federal government had talked to them as well. All of the remains were being routed through Lufkin, which is inside Angelina County, before they were shipped to Barksdale and on to Dover Air Force Base, in Delaware. Washington had decided that the death certificates would be filed in Angelina County. At my father's request, a letter to this effect was faxed to us, officially relieving us of our normal duties of filing the death certificates.

After Dad briefed me on the death certificate situation I brought up the little matter of pay. I wanted to know what we were going to charge for our services.

He shook his head. "No, I've already told them that we're not going to accept any pay for our services."

"Dad, it's the federal government we're dealing with here. It's not like they're strapped for cash."

"It's a matter of principle. We aren't taking any money."

And that was that. There would be no further discussion on this particular subject. At the time, I disagreed with my father, but in the long run I realized he was right—it was a matter of principle.

It was a fine line. I didn't have a problem with people who did profit from the search operation, but our job had been directly related to the actual recovery of the crewmembers themselves. If we had been assigned to, say, delivering body bags out to the sites, we probably would have submitted a bill, but we were given the honor of recovering and transporting these heroes. It wasn't a job; it was a privilege.

* * *

Not long after my father left for home, we received a call from Nacogdoches Medical Center. A patient had passed away and the family had requested our services. Since Nacogdoches is sixty-five miles away, I sent Debi to pick up the body in the '91 hearse so I could stay on call in the county.

Debi had been gone a little over an hour when the Sheriff's Office called. The search teams had discovered another crew-related item. As with yesterday, they wanted me to pick up the item at the Sheriff's Office and take it to Lufkin.

Before I left for the Sheriff's Office, I called Dad to let him know what was going on. He said he would be ready if they called before I returned.

* * *

Just like the day before, I backed into the sally port to receive my precious cargo. Unlike the day before, today I knew where I was going. Not only had I already made the trip, this time Dad had given me much easier-to-follow directions to Dr. Bruce's lab.

A cooler was loaded into the back of the Excursion, as well as a neatly folded body bag. I was told the contents of the body bag were extremely fragile.

Just before we got underway, word came in that the search teams might have located another site. We were put on hold for a few minutes while Terry went into the field to verify this second site. After waiting several minutes, I suggested we go ahead. Dad could take care of the second site if it proved a genuine find. Shane said this would probably save them some time, but might put us on the road for three trips if a late call came in after Dad started for Lufkin. I told him that this would be no problem. We would do whatever was needed.

I went inside the Sheriff's Office and gave Dad another call, telling him he needed to come back into town—they would probably be calling him shortly.

* * *

About twenty minutes after we got underway I heard Dad getting a call on the radio. At this point Dad was really sticking to his word about doing whatever it took to help with the recovery operation. He took the '98 hearse—his baby—into the woods for this removal.

* * *

Nancy Currie was my ride-along astronaut for this trip. She didn't prove quite as talkative as my last rider, but she was certainly every bit as interesting. The hour-long drive seemed to fly by.

When we reached Dr. Bruce's, the two items were placed in "Queen's" care, and I turned around and headed back to Hemphill. I drove as fast as I dared on the slick roads in order to get back into town in case something else came up. However, these two runs would prove to be our only activity of the day.

18

Moving the Nose Cone

ON TUESDAY, permission was obtained from NASA to allow the public to view the nose cone. Reporters and curious citizens alike were led down a short trail from Bayou Bend to view what was the most recognizable portion of the shuttle yet found.

While the public was viewing the nose cone, NASA officials back in Houston, the Incident Command in Hemphill, and the overall operational command in Lufkin were all working on how to go about retrieving this extremely important piece of the shuttle. The first plan was to lift the nose cone out with a helicopter. It would take quite a clearing operation to clear a landing site in the woods. Not only would the trees have to be cleared, but stumps would have to be removed to make a suitable landing area. It was decided that the best plan of action would be to lower a cable to the nosecone from the helicopter. Several trees would still have to be felled in order to prevent the line from becoming tangled, but it wouldn't be a particularly extensive, time-consuming job.

Temple Inland owned the area in which the nose cone had fallen. They allowed the trees to be cut and sent a group to help in any way possible. The actual job of cutting down the trees fell to Felix Holmes, a local longtime U.S. Forest Service employee. He carefully aimed each tree so that it fell away from the site and didn't become entangled with another tree on its way down.

In preparation for the move, workers with the EPA carefully lifted the nose cone from its crater. Once the nose cone was out, it was thoroughly wrapped to prevent further damage while it was in flight.

The recovery team was racing against the clock—or, rather, they were racing against the weather. They needed to get the nose cone out before the cold front moved in. A Blackhawk helicopter generally has very little trouble in rough weather, but there was concern over the heavy load that would be suspended below the chopper. As the cold front approached, another unforeseen problem reared its head. While the storms and rain had yet to develop, the air currents pushing ahead of the front caused the wind to pick up considerably. One look at the rubbery pines swaying in the wind made it clear that there was still a slight chance of entanglement. Felix's clearing would *probably* be wide enough, even with the treetops bending back and forth, but there was still a slim chance that the wind might blow the helicopter just enough for the cable to grab a nearby tree. This was an unlikely occurrence, but one that could endanger the crew of the helicopter and all of the workers and volunteers on the ground in the area. It simply wasn't worth the risk. The helicopter flight was canceled barely an hour before it was to lift off and start toward East Texas.

If the operational command stuck to the helicopter idea, it could be weeks before the weather cleared and nose cone made it out of the piney woods. A change of plans was in order. The leaders decided the nose cone was now to be moved on the ground. The steady coming and going of the workers, the public, and the press over the last two days had already beaten down a path through the brush. On Wednesday afternoon a local businessman was contacted to widen the path with a track hoe. As it turned out, the short path ran through an area covered with mostly young pines, so it took very little time to beat a wide path through the saplings and underbrush.

Wooden pallets were laid end-to-end across a creek that crossed the path about three-quarters of the way to the site. Dirt was mounded up on top of the ends of the pallets to smooth out the surface of the makeshift bridge.

Needless to say, the media was chomping at the bit to get pictures of the effort to move the nose cone. However, removing the barricades at the ends of Bayou Bend would have opened a virtual floodgate. There were already officials and workers from over a dozen organizations working at the recovery site; there was little doubt that the addition of the reporters would have overcrowded the small clearing. DPS public relations officer Greg Sanchez and the Operation's Information Officer Marsha Cooper came up with a compromise. They handpicked three members of the media to accompany them to the site as they stayed out of the way.

A two-and-a-half ton National Guard truck was brought down Bayou Bend to receive the nose cone. This truck was too large to make it down the path, so another mode of transportation was quickly found. In a bit of irony, the government's high-tech Blackhawk helicopter and her well-trained crew had been replaced by a four-wheeler driven by Lin Marcantel. Lin drove a Texas Parks and Wildlife four-wheeler and trailer down the new trail to the site.

Officials from NASA, FEMA, EPA, and employees of Temple Inland looked on as workers for the Texas Parks and Wildlife and the U. S. Forest Service carefully loaded the bundled nose cone onto a steel pallet. A group of workers then lifted the pallet and placed it on the back of the four-wheeler's trailer. Once the pallet was in place, Lin started forward at a slow steady pace while several workers walked alongside the trailer. The three cameramen stayed well in front of the entourage, their cameras flashing away as they took picture after picture of the scene.

Once the nose cone was off the path and onto Bayou Bend, Lin carefully maneuvered the trailer into position behind the deuce-and-a-half. The group of forestry workers once again surrounded the pallet and carefully lifted it off the trailer and into the back of the truck.

From Hemphill the nose cone went straight to Barksdale Air Force Base in Shreveport, Louisiana. From Barksdale, it was taken to Fort Lauderdale, Florida, where skilled engineers had been given the task of piecing the wreckage back together in order to understand just what had gone wrong.

19

The Air Search

GREG COHRS HADN'T been the only local Forest Service Employee asked to take part in the helicopter search on the first day of the shuttle incident. While Greg was on his way to the office in Hemphill, Don Eddings was on his way to meet the Forest Service's contract helicopter at the municipal airport in Pineland. Don arrived at the airport just before the helicopter touched down at the small one-runway field, but the chopper wouldn't be there long. The pilot was warned that a Restricted Flight Area had been declared covering a wide, oblong corridor along the shuttle's path. The airport was just inside the Restricted Area, but the pilot was allowed to return to Lufkin immediately so he wouldn't be grounded at Pineland.

The next day the USFS contacted Washington and gained permission to use their helicopter to assist in the search. By then Greg Cohrs had been assigned to ground search, but Don Eddings was still available.

When Sabine National Forest Ranger Marcus Beard approached Don about performing the air search, Don wasn't sure he was qualified for this job. However, Don had recently received USFS training as a helicopter crew member. A crew member in a USFS helicopter acts a load supervisor and an observer, this training is very thorough and in-depth.

Marcus also brought up another important qualification, "Don, you've been here for forty years. You've peed behind every tree in the county; you probably have a good idea what they look like from above."

* * *

The pilot that the USFS contracted for the operation was certainly more than qualified for the low-level flying that would be required. Brainerd Helicopter Service out of Brainerd, New Mexico, was contracted for the operation, and their pilot, Tracy Armstrong, was sent to the Sabine County area. Tracy had retired from the Army, where he had served as a Blackhawk instructor and as a special ops pilot.

Pilots who make their living flying by the seat of their pants often develop strange superstitions and customs, and Tracy was no exception. When Don first took his seat next to the pilot, he noticed that the pilot was wearing a solid black hood over his face. Only the area around his eyes was visible.

"Why are you wearing that?" Don asked.

The pilot shrugged. "Habit. I've always worn one. I guess it's for good luck."

"Well, if it's for good luck, you wouldn't happen to have one that I could borrow?" Don replied, half joking, and half serious.

Don's concerns grew after they lifted off. Tracy kept the chopper just above the trees as they sped along.

"Don't you think you need to get a little higher?" Don asked.

"No," Tracy flatly replied.

By the end of the first day, Don grew accustomed to the seemingly dangerous low-level flying. He realized that this pilot certainly knew what he was doing.

It didn't take long for Don and Tracy to establish a good working relationship. Tracy moved along the search corridor while Don and two other spotters in the seat behind them searched the trees for debris. Once possible debris was spotted, the chopper was moved over the site and the observers carefully inspected the site and took the GPS coordinates.

During the first two weeks, the primary purpose of the operation was still recovering the shuttle's crew. Since the media was monitoring all radio traffic, Don would not transmit information about potential crew finds over the radio. Instead, since the cell phone couldn't be used in the air because its frequencies could sometimes foul up the helicopter's navigational instruments, Tracy would have to fly to a safe landing location and land in order to inform the command center by cellular phone of their potential important finds.

On Monday, NASA stepped in to help coordinate the helicopter search. Their professional expertise was greatly appreciated. Don was still listed as the Sabine County operation's Air Search Coordinator, but he was also the main observer in the chopper. There was only so much coordinating he could do while taking such an active role in the operation. NASA and the Forest Service Dispatch worked closely with the Operation's Ground Search.

As with the Ground Search, safety was a key issue in the air. Forest Service helicopter operations protocol required the pilot to check in with their coordinates every fifteen minutes—a process called flight following. Tracy wore a timer attached to his leg that was set to go off every fifteen minutes. When the timer buzzed, Don called in the helicopter's coordinates. Should the helicopter suddenly go down without getting a distress call out, the Incident Command Post would know something was wrong when the helicopter couldn't be reached after failing to check in with the coordinates at the proper time. Also, they would have a record of the helicopter's last report; as a result, the search area for the missing helicopter would be more confined.

Tracy's Bell 205 wasn't the only chopper assigned to the recovery operation in Sabine County. A U.S. Army Blackhawk was also stationed at the Pineland airport. Unlike the USFS helicopter, the Blackhawk wasn't actively used for the search— its job was recovery. As soon as Don reported a possible crew or crew-related site, this helicopter would proceed to those coordinates. A canine search team would then be dropped off at the site to find the exact location.

Due to the fact that they weren't involved in the actual recovery, Don's helicopter crew usually didn't even know how successful their day had been until they returned to Hemphill. One afternoon when Don returned to the Incident Command Center he was greeted by several people who seemed unusually glad to see him. Don spotted Terry Lane and asked, "Why is everyone treating me like a long lost brother?"

"You mean no one told you?" Terry asked.

"Told me what?"

"You called in two confirmed crew sites today."

* * *

On the afternoon of Tuesday, February 4, the chopper was flying just above the treetops south of Hemphill. They were searching the Springhill area when Don noticed a pickup parked down an old logging road that ran off of Springhill Road. The pickup passed almost directly underneath them as they flew over.

"Whoa, hold up," Don said.

"What've you got?" Tracy replied as he brought the chopper to a stop.

"There's a truck down there."

While the pilot was trying to position the chopper so Don could get a better view, two people came running out of the woods. The newcomers jumped in the pickup and tore down the road, leaving a cloud of dust.

On Monday the United States Attorney General's Office had released an urgent news brief concerning the looting of space shuttle debris. So far there hadn't been any arrests in Sabine County, but earlier in the week two people had been arrested in Nacogdoches County and the operation leaders had been told to keep a look out for scavengers. Now it seemed as if Don had caught someone red-handed.

Tracy started to give chase, but Don told him to stay where

he was. He didn't think pursuit would be necessary; the logging trail below them was a dead end. If the pickup was going to get out, it would have to come back their way.

Scarcely a minute passed before the truck came tearing back down the road. Using his binoculars, Don tried to inspect the content of the pickup's bed. He saw a round metal object. He made a mental comparison of the debris he had seen thus far and the picture that NASA had shown the people in the operation and decided that this object might be one of the shuttle's circular windows or hatchways. While Don inspected the pickup's bed, Tracy swung the chopper sideways, telling the observer behind him to get the license plate number. However, the pickup rounded the next curve before he could get the entire number. He only had the first couple of digits, and he wasn't one-hundred percent sure about the ones he had. Now Tracy gave chase.

At about the same time the pickup exited the logging road and turned onto Springhill Road toward Highway 83 Don contacted Greg Cohrs at the Incident Command Center. "Greg, we've got one running from us."

"Where are you?"

"Coming out of Springhill Road. He's heading toward Highway 83."

As soon as they were sure the truck was heading for the highway, Tracy flew past the pickup. When the pickup burst out of the dirt road and onto the pavement, the chopper was hovering at the intersection. Still, the flying dust kicked up by the rotor wash prevented the observers from getting the license plate number when the panicked driver turned right toward Hemphill.

Don and Greg both tried to contact someone to stop the vehicle, but, due to the still confusing state of the radio communications, they were unable to find anyone who could help. In fact, when the pickup darted past Bayou Bend, where the Forest Service was just beginning to work on removing the nose cone, there were dozens of patrol cars on either side of the road. The truck sailed right through the middle of scores of

State Troopers.

Once they were past Bayou Bend, the chopper once again flew ahead of the pickup. It was hovering above the road near the Sabine County Hospital, when the pickup came into view.

"He's coming into Hemphill," Don reported.

However, the truck left the Highway, turning right down a dirt road that ran between Highway 83 and Beckham Road.

"No, he's taking the cutoff road beside Dr. Neal's. He'll be coming out at Jay Chance's. Get someone over there."

"Don, is that you?" a voice asked over the radio. It was Brad Bradberry of the Hemphill City Police.

"Yeah. Go to Jay Chance's."

"I'm right here waiting on him."

When the pickup first came around the corner and saw the patrol car parked across the end of the dirt road, it stopped as though the driver was pondering the possibility of turning around and making another break for it. However, the chopper flying overhead proved that there was simply nowhere to hide. Finally, the pickup inched forward and the occupants gave themselves up.

After a few minutes Brad radioed Don and asked if he had seen them pick up anything. Don told him that he thought there might be something in the pickup's bed. There was another long pause before Brad came back on the radio and reported that it was only an old wheel hub.

As it turned out, the suspected looters were only a couple of teenagers. They just wanted to take part in the search and school had prevented them from being part of the organized search, so they formed their own private search team. They swore that they hadn't found a thing and had planned on turning in anything they did find. When they saw the helicopter, they had panicked. Brad informed the teenagers that if they wanted to take part in the search, they needed to report to the Volunteer Staging Area.

* * *

Toward the end of the operation, Sabine County would see another disaster. At around 4:30 on the afternoon of March 27, it was reported that a U. S. Forest Service contract helicopter involved in the Columbia search had gone down east of Farm Road 705 near the San Augustine/Sabine County line. Of the five people on board, two were killed and three were seriously injured. Don and Tracy had completed their tour in the search operation. It was a different chopper, based out of Lufkin instead of Pineland, but Don couldn't help but notice that the two people who had died were sitting in the front two seats—the same seats that he and Tracy had been occupying.

The two men who lost their lives were Charles Krenek, an aviation specialist with the Texas Forest Service, and Jules F. "Buzz" Mier, Jr., a chopper pilot whose Arizona employer had been hired by the U.S. Forest Service to help in the search. The three men who were injured were Matt Tschacher, a USFS employee from South Dakota, Richard Lange and Ronnie Dale, both employees at the Kennedy Space Center in Florida.

20

Reporting on Sabine County

THE RAIN HAD STOPPED coming down in buckets, but it was still drizzling heavily when Laura Krautz's Jeep Wrangler turned off the loop in Nacogodoches and started east on Highway 103. Laura, a reporter for the Tyler Morning Telegraph, followed the approximate path of the shuttle as she passed through San Augustine on her way to Hemphill. Evidence of the disaster seemed to be everywhere she looked that gloomy Thursday morning—mostly in the form of media trucks and numerous official vehicles ranging from the abundance of DPS patrol cars to the occasional bus transporting searchers.

On the way through East Texas, Laura recalled the morning of February 1. Like so many others, the loud rumbling had awakened her from a deep sleep as it shook the roof of her house. Her husband, Larry, a native Californian, had sleepily declared the rumbling an earthquake. However, Laura's father was on the phone in minutes, telling her that the shuttle had fallen apart over Dallas and debris was raining down all over East Texas, including Palestine, which was only twenty miles from their house. "I think they're going to be calling you into work today," her father predicted.

Laura called her boss, and he told her to go to the office, where the assignments editor was already making out plans as to which reporter would go where. She jumped in the shower, changed, and headed to work with her hair still wet. Despite the fact that most of the reporters lived outside of Tyler, they were all at the office within thirty minutes. Laura's heart had hammered away when she first heard that terrible rumbling, and now, five days later, there was still a feel of excitement and exhilaration about being involved in an event that had gripped the attention of the entire United States, if not the entire world.

Laura's Jeep turned right at Ford's Corner in San Augustine County and started toward Hemphill. Unlike so many other reporters, Laura wanted to talk to the people of East Texas and see how this tragedy had affected their lives. She wanted to listen to what the common person had to say and report on the disaster from their perspective. She was already aware that in some ways the cards were stacked against her. The media's normal aggressive style of reporting certainly clashed with the mostly laid-back rural population, and the way the national media often depicted these good people as backwoods hicks certainly hadn't endeared outsiders with cameras and notepads to the country folk.

Once she arrived in Hemphill, Laura's first stop was the city hall. She asked to see the city manager, but he wasn't in. While some portions of the local effort had slowed down this fifth day of the operation, Don Iles was still a busy man and would remain so for quite some time.

Laura's next stop was Starr Funeral Home. Although she wasn't trying to be sneaky, she managed to make it to the front door before my father and I could bolt for the back, which was exactly what we had been doing every time a reporter pulled up in front of the funeral home. At first we were reluctant to give an interview, but when she explained that she wasn't there for explicit details or inside information my father agreed. Dad didn't have the patience to sit and talk to a reporter at the time, so he volunteered me for the interview. However, since a family was coming in shortly to see me about ordering a monument, we scheduled the interview for later that afternoon.

After she left the funeral home, Laura headed back into town. Parking usually isn't a problem in downtown Hemphill. However, on the first Thursday after the shuttle incident, the town was still abuzz with all the temporary residents and curious visitors. Luckily, Laura managed to find someone pulling out of a parking space at the courthouse and she managed to get one of the few spaces close to both the command center and the Sheriff's Department.

Laura grabbed her umbrella and headed for the Sheriff's Department. She asked a few of the deputies and dispatchers for interviews but they dutifully told her she would have to speak with the sheriff, and he was currently at the command center at a news conference.

She left the Sheriff's Department and started toward the command center. Since she wasn't here for the standard news information, however, the news conference didn't interest her in the least. She was hoping to meet a local at the command center who would give her an interview.

After she crossed Main Street, she could see the Fire Hall and the host of reporters outside and about a half dozen news trucks. When Laura turned to start back to the city square a sign outside the Sabine County Visitors Bureau caught her attention—the sign was about finding places to stay. Laura went inside and found Lisa Owens sitting behind her desk talking on the phone. After Lisa got off the phone, Laura asked if there were any rooms available in Sabine County. Lisa replied that the hotels were full and there was a waiting list of hundreds.

Laura then requested an interview and Lisa offered her a seat. Lisa told her how she hadn't been in town on February 1st, but coming back had been strange because of all the new activity. Military vehicles and patrolling helicopters certainly weren't a part of everyday Sabine County life. Before Columbia, Lisa's job had been a relatively quiet one—mostly finding places for fishermen to stay during tournaments. Now she was overwhelmed with the effort to find rooms for all of the searchers, federal workers, and law enforcement personnel who needed a place to stay. The interview lasted about an hour before Laura decided to move on.

She left the visitor's bureau and started back up town, this time on the dual mission of finding an interview and finding something to eat. It was well past noon and she was getting hungry.

She returned to the square and looked around the local shops, finding a place called *Brenda's Talk of the Town*. If there was ever a name of a business that appealed to reporters, this was it. As soon as she walked through the door she was greeted by Brenda Adams, who asked her to sign her guest book. While Laura signed in, Brenda proudly told her that many reporters had come in and signed the book, including some "girls from CNN." Someone brought Laura a soda and offered her a seat. For the first time since she left Tyler, she was able to relax. There were several women in the shop, and all were more than eager to share their experiences. Laura listened with great interest to their friendly chatter.

As much as she was enjoying the group, Laura still had to find something to eat. She asked if they could suggest a good place to eat, and one of the women suggested KC Drugs, which is also on the square. Laura took her leave and once again set off into the rain, which had picked up somewhat since she entered the store.

Laura stepped into the old-fashioned drugstore, walked up to the bar and ordered a chopped beef sandwich to go with the soda she had been given at Brenda's. While she was waiting for her meal, one of the ladies she had just met arrived and ordered lunches for the whole crew back at Brenda's. They talked while waiting for their lunches and before the lady left she gave Laura a hug. Laura was already very impressed by the people here. Hemphill reminded her of the nice little town her grandparents lived in while she was growing up. In a way, it was like going back to a familiar place she'd really never been.

Laura took her sandwich back to her Jeep so she could have a little time to herself before getting back to work. It was only twenty minutes of quiet time, but it was enough for her to gather her thoughts.

Next she returned to Starr Funeral Home. Despite having

already agreed to an interview, she found herself once again explaining that her story was about the people of Sabine County and not the gritty details. After a little good-natured ribbing from my father, she was taken to the arrangement office. She spoke with me for quite some time before taking her leave. It was getting late and she was still supposed to stop by in San Augustine on her way back through.

Laura had wanted five or six interviews in Sabine County and only managed three. However, while she hadn't talked one-on-one with as many people as she would have liked, she felt she had met enough people to give her a good overall feel of the people of Sabine County and the ordeal they were going through. She only hoped she could do the people justice in telling their story.

* * *

The next day, the editors came to Laura. They wanted all the Sabine and San Augustine County stories to blend into one with pictures for a large package to close down their continuing coverage. The story was set to run in the Sunday edition, which would be coming out in two days.

Laura spent all day Friday poring through her notes, listening to her tapes, and sorting through the pictures. The story was about 70 inches of copy when it was completed—the longest story she had ever written. Toward the end of the day, she finally let the story leave her hands.

* * *

On Sunday morning, Laura picked up a paper at a gas station in Tyler. She read the article in her Jeep. It was good—possibly the best story she had ever written. Then, like so many of us, once the work was over the true meaning of the story finally sank in. She returned home and cried.

21

On and Below Toledo Bend

THE FIRST THREE DAYS of the operation focused solely on the ground search. However, a fishing tournament had been taking place on Toledo Bend Reservoir and several fishermen on the lower part of the lake reported being showered with debris. One particularly interesting report was of a piece of debris as big as a compact car that had supposedly splashed down not far from the Texas coastline. There was little doubt that significant portions of the Space Shuttle had disappeared into the murky depths of Toledo Bend Reservoir.

Located on the Texas-Louisiana border, Toledo Bend Reservoir is the fifth largest manmade lake in the United States. The waters of Toledo Bend provide Sabine County with tourism, one of its two primary sources of income (the other major source of income is the timber industry), and half of the population of the county lives along the subdivisions and retirement communities along the lake's shores. The Sabine River Authority is responsible for operating the Toledo Bend Dam and maintaining many of the various parks located along the shores of the lake.

During the first few days of the search, the employees of the Sabine River Authority walked the woods with the other volunteers, participating in the ground search in Sabine County. However, on Tuesday they were called back to Toledo Bend to help with the water search.

Jasper County Sheriff Billy Rowles was the Director of the

newly created Water Search Branch. During his first two days at the helm he had the thirteen-man DPS dive team at his disposal, as well as three divers from Harris County's dive team. During this time, the FBI also brought in high-tech sonar equipment from Miami. On Wednesday, the third day of the water search, a four man team from the Coast Guard joined the search as well.

The all-volunteer Jasper County Emergency Corps also supplied personnel and equipment to assist in combing the shoreline, as well as the depths of Toledo Bend. While they weren't as well equipped as the state and federal organizations, the Jasper County Emergency Corps did have six licensed divers, their own dive boat, and various underwater cameras and search devices.

The first duty assigned to the Sabine River Authority was to search the shoreline for any debris that may have washed ashore. As soon as the water search began, the Toledo Bend Division of the Sabine River Authority had three boats with a crew of three men apiece working their way around the southern portion of the lake. For the most part, little was found during these searches, although they did stumble on an occasional piece of tile that had floated ashore. Still, every inch of the shoreline had to be covered, and the crews worked from sunup to sundown to complete their task.

* * *

On Thursday night Jamie Williams, an employee of the Parks and Recreation Branch of the Sabine River Authority, received a call from his supervisor, Steven Dougharty. Steven told him he was calling the four members of his branch to prepare for a search of Toledo Bend's islands. They were told to dress in thick clothes. It was going to be cold and windy on the lake.

Friday morning the weather was windy with light rainfall. The temperature was in the mid-thirties, but the wind chill combined with the humidity dropped the actual temperature well below freezing. Jeff Wilburn, one of the workers from the

Toledo Bend Division who had been searching the shoreline, was waiting to take the crew out. Four of the five members of SRA's Parks and Recreation Division gathered at the boat ramp and quickly loaded their gear, mostly machetes and some extra food and water. Then, bundled up like Eskimos, Steven Dougharty, James Hopson, Gaylon Eddings, and Jamie Williams loaded into the boat for transportation to Texas Island, the biggest of Toledo Bend's islands.

The only member of the Parks and Recreation Division not present that morning was Gary Parks. Gary has a serious fear of open water and would have steered clear of the boats on the calmest of days. Now, with the lake raging with whitecaps and five foot swells, he would have had to have been bound hand and foot for the rest of the crew to get him in the boat that morning. However, throughout the operation, Gary made up for his inability to help out on the lakes by keeping the boats in constant running order, as well as minding the fort while the other employees were away.

The trip out to Texas Island was a cold, wet one. The cold wind cut like a knife through the extra layers of clothing, and the constant spray of water over the boat's bow kept the four passengers shivering throughout the trip. Although it was relatively short, it seemed a long, grueling ride.

As soon as Jeff beached the boat on Texas Island, the shivering crew jumped to shore and began organizing themselves into a small but efficient search group. The four-man team spread out until there was about ten feet between them. They then started a steady methodical search of the island, combing it back and forth until they had covered every inch of ground. This was no easy task. They used machetes to cut through underbrush that was every bit as thick as the underbrush on the mainland. After the first thirty minutes or so, it also became apparent that the thick clothing that had just barely protected them from the elements on the trip out to the island was now far too hot. As they pressed on, the group began to shed more and more of the heavy clothing, but they were careful to keep track of each item because they knew they would need it for the trip back.

The search of Texas Island proved fruitless. The island was covered with turtle shells from the local turtles that would lay their eggs before dying, as well as beer cans from the local populace who would have their fun on the island, then move on. But there wasn't a single piece of shuttle debris to be found.

Before loading back into the boat, the tired, haggard crew posed while Jeff took their picture. Gripping their machetes tight, the crew looked more mean and ornery than they did tired and weary. This gruff picture would later make its way onto their office wall with a caption under it reading, "If you don't pay in our parks, we will find you."

* * *

Later that same afternoon, Billy Rowles was on his way back to Jasper, listening to the steady traffic on his police radio when he overheard on the radio a distress call from one of the boats on the lake. It was the Jasper Emergency Corps boat. The high waves had begun to wash over the low-sided dive boat.

Billy immediately got on the radio and asked the Incident Command Post to get a chopper out to the boat immediately. With the water as cold as it was, drowning was the least of their worries—a person could easily die of hypothermia in those frigid waters. In fact, only a few months prior to the shuttle incident, the cold lake had claimed the lives of two fishermen.

The Forest Service's helicopter wasn't equipped for such a rescue, but there were a pair of Coast Guard helicopters operating just outside of the area that could more than likely reach the vessel in time. However, these helicopters were monitoring the Coastal Emergency Channel. The ICP was unaware of this and they were unable to contact them using the channels that were being used in the operation. As a result of the miscommunication, there were several terrible minutes when the only vessel that could be routed toward the distress signal was Game Warden's boat, which was still some distance away.

Luckily it turned out that the boat's radio operator had panicked and overreacted to the situation. While there was no doubt that the boat was in danger of being swamped by the high waves, he had failed to take into account the depth of the water, which was barely over a foot where they were at the time. After several tense minutes, the problem was solved by bringing the boat a little closer to land, and then using a bilge pump to get rid of the excess water.

* * *

The searchers on the lake were faced with several difficulties that would severely hamper this portion of the operation. The first and foremost problem was Toledo Bend herself. When the Sabine River had been dammed back in 1966, the lake had filled much faster than had been expected. Instead of taking the years that the engineers had expected, the lake had appeared in only a matter of months, just as had been predicted by locals in the area who knew the Sabine River. As a result of the lake's rapid appearance, the trees hadn't been cleared in time, leaving the lake's surface with a dense array of stumps and the lake's bottom lined with old waterlogged trees that had fallen to the lake's floor. As if this wasn't enough, there were also a number of houses and old cars that had occupied the area when the lake filled, and even some old logging equipment which hadn't been moved out of the way in time. Add to this nearly a half a century of beer bottles and other miscellaneous litter and you have a mess that even the nation's best sonar couldn't penetrate.

At one point, the FBI team decided to test their equipment by dropping two large metal items into the water and watching them descend on the sonar. Even though these items were dropped in full sight of the sonar crew, only one of the items was retrieved; the other was never recovered.

Another factor that would come back to haunt the water search operations was the conditions on the water on the day that the shuttle had gone down. While everywhere else in the county was experiencing a perfectly clear day, there was a thin blanket of fog hanging over the lake. This fog proved to be just enough of a hindrance that it didn't actually block the sight of the falling objects, but it did block out items in the background that might have given the observer a point of reference with which to judge distance. For example, the two men who reported seeing the compact car-sized piece of debris land in the water were fishing in the same area; however, one reported that the item had splashed down within one-hundred yards of their boats, while the other stated it was more like one-thousand yards.

Something else that may have come into play was the speed the debris was traveling. Branch Director Billy Rowles later recalled the sound of 105 millimeter shells as they streaked overhead while he was in Vietnam. Those shells sounded like Mack trucks passing just overhead when they were actually only four inches wide and about two feet long, and were passing well over the treetops. The same could be said as the fishermen heard the roar of items passing by and then saw a tremendous splash made by what may very well have been an item with very little mass but an extraordinarily high velocity.

To make matters worse, even if an item was pinpointed by the sonar teams, it still wouldn't be an easy task for the divers to actually locate it on the lake's bottom. Many of the divers later said that the conditions in Toledo Bend were by far the worst they had ever seen. Not only were there numerous obstacles in the water, but the bottom was mostly silt, meaning the slightest disturbance would cloud the water. And considering the lake's turbulent surface during those first few weeks, there didn't even have to be a disturbance on the bottom for the silt to become churned up. Rarely could a diver see his hand in front of his face.

As the search wore on, various groups of divers came and went with the operation. Around the middle of the second week a group of divers from the Navy arrived in the area. During the first few weeks, not a single item had been retrieved from Toledo Bend, but this lively group decided they would break the deadlock. They offered to buy a keg of beer as a reward to the first team to find a bona fide piece of shuttle debris. It was still several weeks before one of the Houston area dive teams managed to score what appeared to be a piece of the shuttle. Upon further examination it was determined that the item was probably just old scrap metal, but only further tests would tell. In light of only a partial success, the Navy team decided to cough up a partial prize. They bought the Houston dive team a six-pack of non-alcoholic beer.

22
Uncooperative Weather

EAST TEXAS WEATHER is notoriously unpredictable. The cold temperatures and heavy rain that was supposed to blow in on Wednesday remained a mild but steady drizzle all day. However, early on Thursday the bottom dropped out. Just before sunrise, the drizzle turned to a downpour, and the temperature dropped to just above freezing and stayed there.

While planning the day's operation, Greg Cohrs predicted that the weather would play an important factor in the day's search. He imagined it would slow the operation, but he had no idea the weather would continue to worsen throughout the morning, eventually bringing a large portion of the recovery operation to a grinding halt.

* * *

Despite the harsh weather, a large number of determined searchers arrived at the Volunteer Staging Area that morning to receive their instructions for the day. After breakfast, group leaders gave a slightly longer safety speech, warning about the increased danger posed by the harsh weather. The searchers were warned about everything from lightning strikes to hypothermia to twisted ankles due to the slippery condition of the ground.

As soon as the briefings were over, the searchers filed out of the Staging Area. The searchers had come from all over the country and included volunteers from local fire departments, walk-on volunteers from around the country, DPS officers, National Forest Service officials, Texas Parks and Wildlife employees, members of the National Guard, FBI agents, and astronauts. However, when the mass of searchers filed out of the VFW hall, they were all handed yellow rain slickers. Once everyone had on their raincoats it was difficult to tell one group from the next. Even the astronauts in their blue jumpsuits and the DPS officers in their uniforms blended in with the dingy yellow crowd. On the line, everyone was together—we were all part of the same team.

* * *

I hadn't slept at all that night, so, since I was already up, I came to work an hour early. On my way, I took a ride out toward Bronson to kill time. The usually familiar yards and houses lining Highway 184 looked strange. The heavy rain cut visibility considerably, but it couldn't conceal the fact that just about every yard had a small circle or two of yellow police ribbon, marking the location of shuttle debris.

Once I arrived at work I sprawled out on one of the couches in the stateroom next to the office, and, still in my suit and tie, I immediately fell fast asleep. For some reason I wasn't resting well in my own bed, but I had no trouble dozing off once I was at the funeral home. Virginia and Debi came in at eight o'clock, but they didn't wake me until around nine.

For about an hour I wandered impatiently around the office, looking for something to do. At this point, I would have much rather have been in the woods instead of sitting on my hands waiting for a call.

At around eleven o'clock, a UPS package arrived from York Casket Company. A member of Debbie's recovery team had mentioned liking the waterproof tags we were using to mark the body bags, so, late Sunday afternoon I had called York and asked them to send as many nametags as they could get their hands on. I figured these tags could be used by the recovery and the search teams to mark and label not only crew-related items, but debris as well. When I opened the box I saw that York had come through in a big way. The box was stuffed with hundreds of plastic coated nametags.

This gave me my best excuse of the morning to get out of the office. Even better, this gave me an excuse to go to the Incident Command Post. I grabbed the box and started out the door for my car.

* * *

Just south of Hemphill, a long line of yellow clad figures stretched out along the shuttle's flight corridor and began steadily working its way through the woods. The going was rough this morning. Just as the briefings had predicted, the weather had gone from uncomfortable to downright miserable. When they first stepped off the buses, the heavy clothing and raincoats seemed to be adequate to ward off the cold, wet environment. However, the line had only advanced a few feet into the woods before it became apparent that the raincoats weren't made to stand up to East Texas terrain. The briars quickly shredded the thin yellow material. Once the raincoats were torn, the clothing underneath became soaking wet. The volunteer firefighters in their wildland suits were somewhat better equipped, but, after five days of hard use, even these hardy, water-resistant garments were unable to keep the downpour at bay.

* * *

The door to the command center was guarded today, and, when I groped around in my pockets I found I had left my I. D. card at home. Luckily, the state trooper at the door recognized me and let me in.

If the weather was hindering the operation, you certainly couldn't tell by the activity at the command center—it was even more of a madhouse than before. Uniformed State Troopers and Forest Service officials, federal agents in their blue jackets with FBI stenciled on the back, astronauts in their light blue jumpsuits, and National Guardsmen in their camouflage fatigues all mingled together like some sort of themed costume party.

I found Greg Cohrs and asked him where to leave the tags. He directed me to the fire hall's main closet, where the Logistics Section had set up their supplies.

When I made my way across the hall, I was shocked by the number of people I didn't know. Perhaps this wouldn't have been so odd for a person raised in the city, someone who is more accustomed to large crowds of unknown faces, but to be in such a familiar place and only recognize a dozen or so of the close to one-hundred people in the building was a strange feeling for me. And of the few faces I did recognize, most had only become familiar over the last week.

A makeshift desk in the form of a folding table with a rolodex and a file folder was situated in front of the fire hall's storage closet. No one was at the desk, but there was a National Guardsman inside the closet, rearranging the various boxes of rations, batteries, flashlights, and other miscellaneous supplies. When I asked him where to leave the nametags, he told me the person in charge of the supply room was out, but he could take them. As I watched him place the box on a high shelf in the far back I had the feeling that several months from now someone was going to discover a box full of mortuary toe tags and ask, "Where in the world did these come from?" Oh, well, it was no loss, really. The nametags weren't as sorely needed now as they had been on Sunday.

After dropping the nametags off at the storage closet, I wandered around the command center, taking a long look at all the changes that had taken place over the week. A couple of laptop computers and over a dozen phones were scattered about on the oblong table in the back room. Wires crisscrossed the floor, running to numerous phone jacks that had been installed earlier in the week. In the enclosed garage area, portable dividers had been set up, squaring off a large portion of the fire hall into a number of small offices.

One of these makeshift offices drew my attention. The artificial walls in this area were covered with numerous maps of Sabine County. Unlike that enormous first map that was here on the first day, these maps were incredibly detailed—some even appeared to be generated from satellite photos. A narrow corridor, about a mile wide, was present on each of these maps, passing through Bronson, then passing just south of Hemphill, and on to the Six Mile area before exiting into Louisiana just north of the Toledo Bend Dam.

After my brief exploration, I sought out Greg Cohrs and asked if the search teams were making any progress in the woods today. He said the teams had gone out but progress had been so slow that they were probably going to call them in.

When I returned to the funeral home I told Dad that I doubted very seriously we would be called out today, and as it turned out, I was right.

* * *

Thursday's weather conditions had been a major concern of the operation leaders long before the searchers even made their way into the woods that morning. They had taken great pains to see that the searchers were as well-equipped as possible. Logistics Chief Marc Allen had spent the better part of the last two days scrounging up enough raincoats for the entire volunteer portion of the search. When the reports from the field indicated that these raincoats had barely lasted the first fifteen minutes, the leaders at the ICP realized that they might be dealing with a problem that was even greater than they had first perceived. After only an hour, the majority of the volunteers were already drenched to the bone.

It wasn't long before the Incident Commanders and other leaders at the ICP began discussing calling off the search for the day. Everyone seemed to be of one mind on the issue—no one really wanted to postpone the search, but they feared that they might become overly focused on the operation and forget the safety of the volunteers.

The Incident Commanders decided to have a meeting to discuss the matter. All of the upper leadership of the Sabine County operation, several advisors, and a few key individuals were asked to meet at the Sheriff's Office.

While the commanders were gathering, Greg Cohrs called the leaders in the field. He told them that the search might be called off, and asked their opinions on the matter. Although many of the leaders in the field realized the health risks that were involved, several of them were of the opinion that they were already wet and miserable—why not keep going? If some of the woods-worthy team leaders had become so focused that they were oblivious to the danger, then Greg could only imagine the reaction of the common searcher. It certainly didn't help matters that what was appearing to be an inevitable decision seemed destined to be such an unpopular one.

* * *

The leaders in the field halted the line while they waited for a decision. At first, the volunteers greeted the unexpected break with enthusiasm. Many took the opportunity to find shelter under nearby trees and enjoy an early lunch. However, when word made it down the line that the search might be called off due to the weather, the volunteers were furious. Even normally mild-mannered Chip Robberson vented his frustration; with a loud shout, he buried his machete in a nearby pine.

* * *

The Incident Commanders were packed tightly in the Law Enforcement Center's squad room. Everyone realized the wise choice would be to call in the volunteers, but no one wanted to be the one who pulled the plug on the operation. Everyone present was greatly relieved when Safety Officer Brad Moore spoke up, saying what was on everyone's mind, "I really think we need to shut down the volunteer part of the search."

Everyone agreed. They decided to call in the volunteer searchers, but leave the National Guard units in the field, since they were much better prepared to handle the elements.

All of the phone lines at the sheriff's office were tied up, so Greg stepped outside to place the call to the leaders in the field. Perhaps it was just his imagination, but when he stepped out into the rain, it seemed that the downpour let up. It would certainly look awful if they called in the volunteers and the rain suddenly quit. However, the decision had been made, so Greg made the call.

* * *

As soon as the Forest Service leaders flagged the line to show where the day's search had stopped, the search teams set out toward their new pickup point, which was to be the clearing down Fire Tower Road. This was the same clearing where Debbie's FBI team had gathered on Sunday morning, before setting off on four-wheelers for the first recovery of that day.

When the ragged volunteers began to emerge from the woods, Raybon Waller's covered carport came into view—shelter at last. The trudging line started picking up speed until many were in a dead run for the shelter. Laughter rang out during this comical mad dash through the rain. For a while, at least, the upbeat feeling among the searchers had returned.

However, after an hour of waiting under the crowded shelter for the buses to arrive, the grumbling returned in force. It would still be some time before the wet, agitated searchers were taken back to the VFW Post, and, when they arrived, they were told that the National Guard had been allowed to continue their search. This added a touch of jealousy to the matter—a feeling of "if they're out there, why aren't we?"

Greg's perception that the weather was letting up proved incorrect. The downpour continued and, if anything, it grew worse throughout the afternoon. For the volunteers, however, this was beside the point; they wanted to be out in the woods doing their part to complete the mission. The determination of the volunteers was such that they would just about do anything to complete the mission at hand. However, the leadership was still fully capable of taking a step back, realizing what had to be done for the safety of those involved, and make the correct, albeit unpopular, decision. The operation had the best of both worlds, determined workers and intelligent leadership.

23
The Expanding Operation

T
HE WEATHER IMPROVED somewhat by Friday morning. It was still raining, but it was no longer coming down in buckets. The conditions were still cold and wet. The ground was slick with mud, and the creeks were swollen from yesterday's rainfall; many of these creeks would have to be waded by searchers throughout the day. Still, despite the bad weather, the volunteer portion of the search remained in the field throughout the day.

With almost a full week under its belt, the organization of the search was rapidly maturing. Some of the local volunteers who had been in the line since the first day were beginning to drop out due to fatigue, illness, and the need to get back to their jobs. However, the volunteers coming from out of town had kept the number of volunteers in the line fairly stable throughout the week. As of Friday, there were still six Forest Service led search groups. These volunteer teams numbered about 25 to 35 apiece, for a total of around 175 searchers.

Of course, by the end of the first week, the volunteer portion of the operation actually made up less than half of the searchers involved. On Friday morning another National Guard unit, including a group with the National Guard Signal Corps arrived, swelling the Guard presence to about 230 searchers. A group of fifteen mounted officers with the Texas Department of Criminal Justice group were searching a portion of the Indian Mounds Wilderness area north of the Indian Mounds Recreation Area where debris had been reported by fishermen to have fallen into the lake and crashed into the timber; this area was just north of the shuttle's debris path. Eighty Native Americans, members of national fire suppression crews from Oklahoma, had also played an important role in the search since the middle of the week. Thirteen two-to-three-person response teams, made up of local police assets and Forest Service officials, were busy answering calls throughout the county. Including the FBI assets, the DPS dive teams, and all the other organizations involved, there were about 650 people involved in the Sabine County recovery effort.

The day's search progressed quite well. Several important pieces of debris were located and tagged with GPS, but there were still no new crew-related sites and two of the crewmembers were still unaccounted for. All in all, the day was a success, but the mission would not be considered a *complete* success until the last astronaut had been returned home.

Late Friday afternoon Greg Cohrs and Jamie Gunter sat down to prepare the plans for the next day's search. During the course of the day, the Incident Commanders had been approached with an offer to increase their manpower by one-thousand additional searchers over the weekend, an increase that would almost triple the searchers operating in Sabine County. This offer had been the subject of much debate, but in the end it was decided that this dramatic increase would overwhelm the local leadership and logistical assets. How would these newcomers be fed, housed, and transported to and from the woods? Besides, the commanders imagined that they would be working with a slightly larger workforce Saturday anyway. Most of the command, the field leaders, and the government resources, such as the National Guard, the FBI, and DPS, would remain the same; however, they looked for a large increase in the number of walk-on volunteers. Word of the massive volunteer turnout had spread throughout the nation and many people like Chip Robberson had come from far away to help in the recovery operation. Greg and Jamie imagined that many of the helpers that hadn't been able to come during the week would take advantage of the weekend and drive to East Texas to lend a hand. While this was nowhere near the one-thousand that had been offered, even this small increase would lead to some revisions in the current plans and add an additional workload to the local leadership assets, which were already stretched thin. Search teams would have to be restructured, and if enough volunteers arrived, more teams would have to be organized.

Work on the new plan was well underway, yet far from finished, when Terry Lane came into the room at about 8:45 that evening. He told Greg that he was needed at the Emergency Operations Center in Lufkin, immediately.

"Am I under arrest?"

Terry laughed. "No, but it's an urgent planning meeting. They want a progress report from this region and I've been instructed to get you there."

Greg said he was busy and asked if the trip could be put off for another hour or so, at least until Saturday's plan was complete.

Terry replied that time was of the essence. The incident commanders in Lufkin wanted the meeting to begin as soon as everyone arrived, and Hemphill was the farthest ICP involved in the meeting.

Greg quickly completed his necessary work and transitioned the planning information over to Jamie, who took over the remainder of the task of planning Saturday's schedule. Greg then gathered the maps and documents he figured would be important for the upcoming report.

Marcus Beard overheard the conversation about sending Greg on a flying trip to Lufkin and he balked at the idea. Greg had been working an average of sixteen intense, high-stress hours a day since the operation began. Terry said that they had wanted the Ground Search Coordinator's input at the meeting, but he also understood the strain the leaders in the Sabine County ICP had been working under. He was sure Lufkin commanders would understand if Greg was too tired to make the meeting. However, Greg insisted on making the trip. Like the rain-soaked volunteer searchers who on the previous day had put their own health out of their mind in order to push forward with the operation, Greg insisted he was okay. Yesterday morning the searchers had been saying that they were already wet and cold, how could their condition get any worse? Now Greg was basically saying he was already tired, what would a few more hours without sleep hurt? Besides, Terry would be driving and he was under strict orders to deliver Greg to the meeting and then ensure his safe delivery after the meeting.

* * *

It was around ten-thirty when Terry and Greg first arrived at the Lufkin Civic Center. The Civic Center had been converted to an office building and was full of office cubicles. There were phone lines and cables running throughout the halls, and, even though it was late at night, there were still a large number of people working and milling around. The nighttime skeleton crew in Lufkin was an impressive array of manpower when compared to what was being used in Sabine County.

"If we had all these people and resources, we'd be done by now," Greg jokingly commented to Terry as they walked down the hall toward the meeting.

When they reached the meeting room, they weren't exactly sure what to expect. And they weren't sure why this briefing was to be given in person, rather than over the phone or by fax; everyone knew Jerry Kidd's Planning Section was doing a great job of keeping the upper command in Lufkin abreast of the situation, and each evening Greg had been sending updated maps of areas searched during the day. Of the thirty some odd people in the room, Greg and Terry recognized several who had been working in Sabine County over the last week. Aside from Terry, there were three other FBI agents who had been working out of the area—Ed Lueckenhoff, Pete Galbraith, and Shane Ball. Also familiar were Brent Jett and John Grunsfeld, two of the astronauts at the meeting. Captain Paul Davis and Sergeant

Michael Bradberry with the Texas DPS were also in attendance, as were several familiar faces with the Texas Forest Service.

Since Terry and Greg were the last to show, the meeting started as soon as they arrived. Greg had no sooner taken a seat than Astronaut James Wetherbee, the NASA official presiding over the meeting, asked him to tell them what Hemphill was doing in the search effort. Greg took the map he had brought with him and indicated the areas that had been searched and spoke briefly about what they were finding and how the search was progressing.

When Greg finished, Wetherbee asked why they weren't picking up shuttle debris as they found it. Greg replied that since the five crewmembers had been recovered in Sabine County, they believed the other two would be in the area. He told the group they were focusing their efforts on locating and recovering the remaining crewmembers. He explained that the search was being conducted as a grid-search with searchers from two to twenty feet apart and shuttle debris finds were flagged, GPS'ed and inventoried.

"Okay, thank you," Wetherbee said. He seemed satisfied with the answer, but he wasn't exactly enthusiastic.

When Greg took his seat he had a sinking feeling that he had somehow not presented the case well enough and the Sabine County resources were going to be diverted elsewhere.

Greg even found himself wondering if the protection of the dignity of the crew of Columbia might actually do them harm here tonight. Out of respect for the crew and their families, discussion about recovery of crewmembers had been suppressed. The most sensitive part of the operation was taking place in Sabine County, and it was proceeding without song and dance for the media. The Incident Commanders were keeping the upper Command up to date, and Jerry Kidd's Planning Section and Marc Allen's Logistics Section were doing an excellent job of keeping up with all the required reports, but it was conceivable that the lack of outward communication with the public at large could cause the upper command—which was operating sixty miles away in Lufkin—to misunderstand what was really going on in Sabine County.

Next San Augustine was asked to present their operation. An FBI agent who was Greg's San Augustine counterpart stepped forward. The operation in San Augustine was similar to the one in Sabine County, but there were differences. Both groups were searching inside an established corridor, but they were going about it in very different ways. The Sabine group was searching along either side of the projected centerline of the corridor and moving outward toward the edges, while the San Augustine group was searching in patches in sort of a jigsaw puzzle pattern, near known debris sites. Both methods had their pros and their cons. In short, the San Augustine method had the potential to yield quicker results since it focused on known patches of debris. However, the San Augustine method was less efficient overall. It would be very difficult to complete, since they would have to go back and fill in all the irregular spaces between the patches.

Greg wasn't sure if they had already decided the course of action before the meeting or if Wetherbee was simply a very decisive individual—as soon as San Augustine's report was finished, the astronaut rose from his chair and made his decision. There was no committee discussion, or any hesitancy. The people from Sabine County were told that the lion's share of this weekend's assets would be coming to their area. Even resources already operating in San Augustine County would be redirected to Sabine County. The recovery of the astronauts was still the top priority, and they were sending as much help as possible to the area most likely to make the final two recoveries.

Wetherbee then asked Greg if there was anything specific that would be needed to make Saturday work. Dozens of items popped to mind, such as transportation, food, and lodging, but Greg only asked for the most crucial item—experienced woodsmen to serve in leadership roles in these new teams.

Wetherbee turned to two of the Texas Forest Service officials present, Mark Stanford and Paul Hannemann and asked if he could help remedy this situation. Paul said he would see what he could do.

After the meeting Terry drove Greg back to Sabine County. They arrived back in Hemphill at one in the morning. They would have only a few hours sleep before the preparations for the next day's search began.

* * *

On Saturday morning, Greg went to the U. S. Forest Service Office early in order to get a head start on the hectic day ahead. Together with Paul Dufour, a U. S. Forest Service Timber Sales Specialist whom Ranger Beard had provided to assist Greg, they began making several copies of the maps of search assignments to give to the search teams. At this point, Greg was unsure how many people would be arriving as a result of last night's meeting, but he knew the operation would be dealing with much more than they had planned the night before. The only way to tackle the problem would be to reorganize the groups after the briefing. This meant it would take more time to get the groups into the woods, but this delay was simply unavoidable.

The day didn't exactly get off to a glorious start. For quite some time Greg and Paul were locked in a struggle with a malfunctioning copier. By the time they were able to get all the extra maps copied, they were running late.

When the two men arrived at the VFW Post, they were shocked to see cars lined all along the shoulders of the road. The parking lot was even worse; the cars were packed like sardines. Even the rodeo's parking lot next door was filled with DPS patrol cars. Greg made the mistake of turning into the VFW hall parking lot, hoping beyond all hope that a parking space might be available—no such luck. He was forced to turn out of the parking lot, and drive back down the road a quarter of a mile in order find a parking space along the shoulder.

Carrying stacks of maps, the two men alternated between jogging and a brisk walk as they made their way along the shoulder of Highway 184 and then across the VFW post's parking lot. As they approached the door, they began to run into large numbers of people standing outside; this seemed strange. When Greg opened the door into the Volunteer Staging Area, the sight took what little breath he had left right away from him. The volunteers weren't just seated in chairs and lined against the wall; they were packed shoulder to shoulder throughout the room.

* * *

That Saturday morning the Sabine County operation had received even more searchers than the one-thousand they had turned down the day before. There were now seventy agencies, groups and volunteer organizations, not to mention almost two-hundred walk-on volunteers. All told, the six-hundred or so people who had been working out of the county had swelled to 1828 overnight.

Although the actual planning for today's search wouldn't begin until Greg and Paul arrived, the Incident Command leaders were already hard at work organizing the searchers.

A key player in this early morning organization was Planning Section Chief Jerry Kidd, of the Texas Forest Service. Greg would later say that, while he was exhausted and almost stretched to his limit on this day, Jerry, who had the benefit of a little more rest, was at his best that Saturday morning. Jerry regularly taught classes on the Emergency Management System, so he simply put his working knowledge to use. The chief ingredient in the Emergency Management System is the organization of assets, so Jerry immediately set to work doing what he could to put as much organization into the morning's chaos as possible. Each of the six teams that had worked yesterday were asked to take their place at certain tables near the walls of the VFW hall. All of the newcomers were asked to congregate in the center of the post, remaining close to the group they came with. While there was no way of knowing how the groups would be divided for today's search until the actual planning was underway, Jerry's initial preparations would speed the process once the ball was rolling.

Another important concept Jerry taught in his classes was the theory of "Divide and Conquer," meaning that a monstrous task was easier to handle once it was broken down into several smaller tasks. To meet this end, the National Guard units were kept where they could be instructed separately. The newly arrived units were told to join the old units behind the rodeo arena where they would receive their instructions as soon as possible. Also, the Texas Department of Public Safety force of 226 troopers and ten officers were sent to the rodeo arena where they would be briefed separately.

Jerry was not alone in these early morning preparations. All of the Incident Command Leaders, the local organizational leaders, and the leaders of the newly arrived groups and organizations were busy that morning. No one knew where they would be assigned for the day, but everyone knew their place for receiving their instructions.

Thus there was an underlying order already in place when Greg arrived in what seemed to be complete chaos. Still, it was going to take some time to get these groups organized and into the woods.

* * *

The volunteers were packed into the hall like cord wood stacked on end. Now it was easy to understand why a lot of people had been milling around outside. There was literally no place to stand or walk in the large VFW Hall. Greg pushed through the crowd constantly repeating "Excuse me" as he made his way toward the stage at the other end of the hall. As luck would have it, one of the persons he bumped into on the way was his son, Adam, who had returned from Lamar University in Beaumont to volunteer for the weekend. Adam had been frustrated all week because he had not been able to help with the search; he felt a special bond with NASA because of his participation in the Texas Aerospace Scholars Program. They exchanged a quick hug and Adam wished his father luck before Greg pressed on toward the stage.

As soon as Greg reached the head of the crowd, he was rushed up to the podium. Tired from lack of sleep and still in a state of shock at the tremendous number of people present, Greg stammered his way through his operational portion of the morning briefing. Several times he had to stop and step to the side to ask a question or two before proceeding. However, with the help of Jerry and Paul, Greg was able to cover all the important details. His weariness was beginning to show, but he was still fully capable of getting the job done. After Greg finished the Operations portion of the briefing, he turned the podium over to Brad Moore for the safety briefing.

Once the briefing was over, the operation's leaders started organizing the day's search. DPS Sergeant Michael Bradberry was given the task of dividing the DPS assets, reinforcing the existing teams with small groups of troopers, and then creating a team made up entirely of DPS personnel. Ed Lueckenhoff, an Assistant Special Agent in Charge out of the FBI Dallas Field Office, saw that the FBI's assets were divided among the teams. Jerry contacted the extra transportation that would be needed and soon had extra buses en route from the local schools. He and Brad Moore also saw that the new medical assets that had arrived were properly distributed so they could respond to any injury that might take place along the line.

As for the forestry experts that would be needed to work the compasses and GPS units, Paul Hannemann managed to come through despite having only a few hours in the middle of the night to work with. He and Bill Rose, also of the Texas Forest Service, contacted several consulting foresters in the area and secured their services. The foresters with superior navigational skills were distributed among the newly formed groups, and there were enough personnel left over to form yet another search team.

Despite the leadership's best attempts to organize the search, the massive influx of newcomers did present a problem. Delays were inevitable. Over the course of the week, the morning routines had become shorter as the people involved began to learn their roles in the operation. Yesterday it had taken an hour to get the teams into the woods. Today it took two and a half hours. When Greg later asked Adam how things had gone with his search that day and expressed his frustration about the length of time it had taken to get the search teams to the field, Adam said, "Dad, I thought it was pretty fast considering all the people that were there." By the time the searchers hit the woods most of the incident leaders were exhausted, and the day had hardly begun.

* * *

The weekend also saw the beginning of several changes in the local operation's command structure. Many of the Incident leaders who would be taking over various posts during the second week arrived early in order to familiarize themselves with the operation. Mark Ruggiero of the USDI Fish and Wildlife Service was going to be brought in as a third Incident Commander for the second week. The reasoning behind this move was that his experience in the incident command system— he had served as incident commander for several forest fires and disasters—would serve as an asset when combined with the local knowledge of the current commanders.

Another change took place in the Operations Section. Jamie Gunter was rotated out as Operations Chief and replaced by the joint leadership of Ronnie Hamm and Steve Weaver. Jerry Kidd also received assistance in the Planning Section with the addition of Co-Section Chief Red Anderson.

While several changes were in the making, some positions remained the same. The two initial incident commanders, Billy Ted Smith and Sheriff Tom Maddox, were retained as co-incident commanders. Greg also continued to plan and direct the search as Ground Search Branch Director, with the only real difference being that the search area was formally divided into Divisions along logical, identifiable boundaries and Division Supervisors were assigned to improve span of control. Many of the outgoing supervisors also remained at the ICP post for several days to serve in both official and unofficial roles as advisors to their former positions.

Despite the chaos of the weekend, these additions and changes were made smoothly and efficiently. The Incident Command System provided specific instructions on how to go about these changes in command, enabling the leadership to be altered without skipping a beat. The joint commands were somewhat out of the ordinary, but, given the fact that they were dealing with an operation that was even more complex than the World Trade Center cleanup, these extra leaders were necessary to allow the Commanders, Chiefs and Branch Directors to fulfill their duties. The system proved flexible enough to allow for these irregularities without hindering the operation in the least.

These smooth transitions were also a tribute to the operation's leadership. There was little room for individualism and certainly no room for jealousy in this complex operation. They had to work as a team if they were going to be successful.

* * *

That night, the leaders sat down to make the operational plans for the following day. They figured they wouldn't have quite as many workers on Sunday as they had on Saturday. For one thing, they knew that many of the weekend volunteers would probably call it quits after the first hectic day. The plan was structured around using the same number of search teams, but with fewer people in each group. In a way, this might prove as much an asset as a liability, since the smaller groups would be easier to manage. The next morning their prediction proved correct. There were only a little over thirteen hundred volunteers, around five hundred less than the day before.

Indeed, Sunday proved much easier to manage than the

day before. For one thing, the routine had been established—everyone knew what to do and where to go. However, they were still dealing with twice the number of people they had worked with during the week. It still took almost two hours to get the searchers into the woods, but the process was much smoother with less confusion than the day before.

The weather remained cold, never getting above 44 degrees, and the showers returned, although it wasn't the steady downpour that had been experienced on Thursday. Some of the newcomers began to worry that the search might be called off again, but the veterans knew better; it had rained harder than this on Friday morning and they had stayed out.

All in all the day proved a success, but, once again, there was no sign of the two remaining crewmembers.

* * *

By Monday morning, Greg felt the weekend had been a mixed blessing. The extra searchers had certainly allowed more ground to be covered, but there was concern about some of the area searched because of the difficulty of keeping fifty to eighty searchers organized in an effective grid line. Normal span-of-control is about five persons per supervisor with most fire crews having a crew boss, three squad bosses, and three squads of six, for a total of about twenty persons. The reduced search teams would be much closer to this more efficient number.

Greg felt Monday morning's briefing and the following preparations went much smoother than the day before. However, Monday morning did bring new changes to the operation's leaders. For one thing, the school day created a shortage of buses. It also turned out that the DPS decided to rotate every one of their nearly 300 personnel on that day, meaning that a considerable amount of experienced personnel had been replaced by newcomers and all of them had to be assigned to particular groups. Also, the Sabine County operation now had to shoulder the additional task of recovering debris. Still, the search teams were loaded onto the buses that were available and relayed into the woods with a minimum of confusion. Despite the day's difficulties, and the fact they were still dealing with about twice the number of searchers as they had during the first week, the leaders in Sabine County were well on their way to returning to the efficiency they had reached by the end of the first week.

24
Feeding the Masses

BELINDA GAY'S KITCHEN crew at the VFW worked almost nonstop during the first week of the operation. Many of those involved actually began staying overnight, sleeping on rough cots in the back of the building. By the weekend, it still wasn't apparent how long the local crew would be in charge of the kitchen, but it was apparent that they couldn't keep this break-neck pace forever.

During the first week other groups that were helping in the kitchen alternated coming in to help. Some of these groups were from the local churches, and some were simply neighbors and friends who had come together to form an impromptu cooking team. The kitchen also received help from many of the local searchers who had become too physically exhausted to continue the search in the woods but still wanted to help in some way. Another very important group of volunteers were those from the established volunteer organizations, such as the American Red Cross and the Salvation Army.

While there certainly wasn't a lack of volunteer assistance, Belinda was still trying to keep herself and her original cooks as the core team at the Volunteer Staging Area, in order to utilize their experience. By the second week, she decided that they needed to make a schedule before they wore themselves ragged. The original cooks were organized into two teams that would alternate coming in to cook every other day.

It was an odd change. The cooks certainly needed the rest, but, in a way, they felt guilty and restless while they were away from the kitchen and actually found themselves wanting to come back to help.

There were other changes in the kitchen throughout the beginning of the first week and on into the second week. Now that the eyes of the nation were focused on Sabine County, food and assistance began arriving from everywhere. Much like the household cooks in Sabine County who had been bringing food from their own kitchens, many of these generous donations of food came from individuals. There were incidents of people actually driving several hours just to bring a casserole dish to the Volunteer Center.

On Thursday, February 6, a group from Gregg County arrived with a portable kitchen. This proved to be one of the greatest additions to the Volunteer Staging Area. Throughout the second week, the Gregg County cooks prepared all of the meat products for breakfast, lunch, and supper. Their kitchen prepared everything from fried chicken to sausage gumbo.

Now that there wasn't such a pressing need at the VFW, many of the local volunteers who had been bringing food to the Staging Area turned their attention elsewhere. Plates of food were prepared in local kitchens and taken to the dispatchers, officers who were on duty, and anyone else who was unable to leave their post in order to go out to the VFW hall and eat. It was an unwritten priority among the people of Sabine County to see that everyone was given a good meal.

People from all over East Texas donated more than just their food and cooking expertise—some donated items that were in need in the kitchen. For instance, Dr. Grover Winslow, Hemphill's longtime physician, loaned a large steamer from Twitty's, his local restaurant. Many of the local grocery stores, including Brookshire Brothers and the Wal-Mart stores in Jasper and Many, offered necessary items at greatly discounted prices. Even organizations with no direct local ties pitched in: at one point a freezer full of Blue Bell ice cream was donated to the Sabine County VFW hall.

Volunteers also assisted in such seemingly insignificant, yet very important, tasks as cleaning and running errands. One such cleaning volunteer, who achieved near legendary status among the kitchen crew, was Glenda Keel. Always a lady, Glenda would often arrive at the VFW post wearing heels and a dress. With her cleaning supplies carried in a small bucket, she would proceed directly to the building's two bathrooms. Once inside she would give each bathroom a cleaning that could pass even the most vigorous inspection. However, what really impressed the ladies in the kitchen was that, despite the fact that these bathrooms were usually filthy from the use of hundreds of searchers and volunteers, Glenda always looked every bit as proper when she left as she did when she arrived. Somehow, she always managed to clean the filthy bathrooms without getting so much as a smudge on her.

* * *

After the first few days, officials from the office of the Surgeon General arrived. Among other duties, they assumed the important job of overseeing the quality of food. This job was undoubtedly very crucial to the health of the searchers, especially considering how many cases of diarrhea had been reported in those first few days. However, their new role didn't always endear these newcomers to the local cooks. Understandably erring on the side of caution, the inspectors vetoed many of the foods that had been prepared in the local homes, ordering them to be thrown away.

In most cases, this simply caused some grumbling, but the cooks did as they were instructed and the questionable food was deposited in the trash. However, there was at least one instance of a minor underground rebellion. One of the most popular local food items brought to the Volunteer Staging Area was homemade preserves and jams. When the government officials stepped in, they immediately instructed the cooks to use only store-bought preserves and jams; the rest was to be disposed of. This didn't exactly set well with the searchers when they came in the next morning. As it turned out, the cooks on duty that day had the foresight not to throw away the homemade preserves; they simply hid them in the kitchen cabinets. When the complaints started coming in, they solved the dilemma by taking the preserves out of their jars and placing them in bowls that were then taken out to the tables. When the inspectors asked about the bowls, the cooks simply said that they had taken store-bought jelly and placed it in bowls for easy access. Either the ruse worked, or the inspectors chose to look the other way. Given the fact that there is no such thing as Welch's "Mayhaw Jelly," the latter is probably the case.

* * *

Near the middle of the second week, the local cooks found out that their role in the food unit would be winding down. Starting the third week, the government would be taking over the food distribution entirely. Having just started their new schedule, the cooks felt as though they were just now really getting into the swing of things.

Due to VFW regulations, a member of the post has to always be present while the post is open; even if it is rented out. This meant one person, usually Belinda or Roger, remained with the food unit throughout each day even after the new cooks arrived. However, this was only an honorary role; the local cooks were now out of the kitchen. This absence of local help in the kitchen left a void within the community. It had felt so good to be a part of something so noble, and now it appeared as if the operation we had helped create was beginning to outgrow the need for local help.

25
Back to Work

THE BAD WEATHER continued to hinder the search for the remaining crewmembers. Despite the influx of almost one-thousand searchers, only one crew-related item was found late Saturday afternoon. Dad made this one trip to Lufkin late Saturday night. Otherwise, everything had been quiet since Wednesday.

The operation really picked up steam on Monday morning. The entire town was bustling with renewed energy as soon as the rains let up. However, Starr Funeral Home was an exception to this increase in activity. Not only had everything been quiet with the shuttle recovery, but things were slow at work as well. While everyone else was getting a fresh start that Monday morning, we were once again stuck in the office, twiddling our thumbs, waiting for the phone to ring. The boredom and anxiety finally got to my father; he went home early that afternoon. Due to his early departure, he wasn't at the office when I received a call from the sheriff's office.

The search teams had discovered one of the two remaining crewmembers through their systematic grid search. I was given brief directions over the phone and told to drive straight out to the scene. The directions were easy enough; the site was less than a mile from my father's house.

As soon as I was off the phone, I called Dad to see if he wanted to meet me at the site. He wasn't home. I imagine if I had been stuck making a recovery by myself on the first couple of days I would have been nervous as hell, but last week seemed years behind me.

* * *

I flew down Highway 87, but not long after I exited off onto Farm Road 2928 I eased up a little so I could watch for the site. About a mile down the road I saw several cars parked on the shoulder. A large white van towing a small white trailer was parked among the vehicles.

The van didn't have identifying markings, but I knew it belonged to one of the FBI's recovery teams. Dad told me that he had worked with a fourth FBI recovery team Saturday and that this team carried their equipment in just such a vehicle. He wasn't quite as impressed as he had been with Debbie's group, but he said they were a very thorough team.

I parked the Excursion just ahead of the cars and got out. I could see one Humvee parked about a hundred feet into the woods and another that was parked right at the edge of the trees. A group of National Guardsmen taking a break at the closest Humvee were the only people to be seen at the site. Everyone else was in the woods.

As I made my way over to the first Humvee, a man in an FBI recovery t-shirt stepped out of the woods, and also started walking in the direction of the group of soldiers. I made my way over to him and said I was there to help with the recovery of the crewmember. He told me he would let the person in charge know I was here—I assumed he meant Terry—and directed me to wait by the Humvee until he came for me.

The FBI agent spoke to an officer at the vehicle, and then returned to the woods. I remained behind. Waiting was certainly something that I was growing accustomed to.

While we waited, a two-seater ultralight aircraft droned slowly overhead. Neither the soldiers present nor I were aware that these pilots were part of the search and recovery efforts. We assumed the media had found a loophole around the no-fly regulations. One of the soldiers turned to the officer and jokingly asked permission to open fire. The officer laughed and replied that if they had brought their weapons they would. I offered to return to the Excursion and get the pistol out of the glove box, but I doubted I could hit it. You know you're in East Texas when a citizen is better armed than the National Guard.

It was a good thirty minutes before another FBI agent stepped out of the woods and started our way. I walked to meet him.

I asked if Terry was still in the woods.

"Terry who?"

"Terry Lane."

"No, he's not here."

That blew my mind. Terry had been so omnipresent over the last week that it never dawned on me that a recovery could take place without him. "Oh, who's in charge of this site?" I asked.

He paused. "You mind if I ask what agency you're with?"

"I'm with the local funeral home. We've been helping with the recoveries."

"Do you have any I.D.?"

Actually, my father and I had been provided with I.D. badges on the first day of the operation, but these temporary laminated cards supplied by the Jasper Fire Department had never been replaced with the new cards FEMA had given out half way through last week. My card was outdated, so I'd left it at home. However, I didn't even get my mouth open with a reply before one of the Guardsmen at the Humvee said, "I'll vouch for him."

I didn't realize it at the time, but one of the group standing there with me was John Whitten, a local man from Pineland. I hadn't recognized him in his fatigues. In fact, I didn't even know he was in the National Guard.

The agent nodded at the Guardsman; then turned back to me. "Sorry about that."

"No problem," I said. "Do you need me to follow you back in or stay where I'm at?"

"Just hang tight for right now."

No sooner had he said this than a third agent popped out of the woods and started toward the team's white van.

The first agent pointed at the newcomer and said. "Ask him where he needs you. He's over the site."

I left the second agent and started toward the van. I caught up with the agent in charge of the site as he exited the van carrying a folded white body bag. I told him who I was and asked what he needed me to do.

"Who called you out here?" he asked.

"The command post," I replied. I wasn't exactly sure who I had spoken with, but I knew where the order originated.

"I thought you were supposed to pick up at the Sheriff's Department."

"That's the way we've worked some of the recoveries; I've helped at the sites on others. Just tell me what you need me to do."

"Go back to town. We'll call you when we need you to pick up there."

"Okay, I guess I could do that," I agreed, but I was a little hesitant. On Tuesday one of the agents at a site had sent us back to town and it turned out that it wasn't exactly what the command center had in mind. I wanted to avoid any confusion on this, my first solo call out to a scene. "Are you sure you don't want me to stay? I won't mind waiting at the road if that's what you need me to do."

"No," he replied. He gave a quick nod at the Excursion, "That thing draws too much attention."

I glanced at the big white FBI recovery van, but didn't say a word. "Do you want me to leave my jump cot?"

"Your what?"

"The collapsible stretcher we've been using to make recoveries in the woods. It's a lot easier than carrying the body bags."

"I don't think we'll need it. We've got enough people to help carry it out."

"How about body bags?" I nodded at the bag in his hand. "I've got heavy duty bags in the Excursion."

"No, thank you," he replied stiffly.

I didn't catch the cold tone. Unaware that I was treading on his toes, I pressed on, trying a little too hard to be helpful. "We ordered the bags for y'all. You're more than welcome to them. They'll do a lot better in the brush than those you've got."

"I think we got it under control. We're putting the remains in one body bag and then placing that bag inside another."

This time I caught the tone. "Oh, well, that certainly ought to work," I said with the friendliest smile I could muster. "I didn't think of using two of them."

Apparently the agent didn't feel like taking the extended olive branch. "Yeah, well, we've done this before," he said coolly, then turned and left before I could reply or apologize.

* * *

I didn't go back to the funeral home when I returned to town. Instead, I went by the Sheriff's Office and stayed there, talking with the dispatchers.

About a half an hour later I saw Shane talking to an agent in the parking lot, so I stepped outside to see if he had any news on the Six Mile site. As soon as he saw me, he said, "I thought you were out at the site."

"They sent me back."

He gave me a questioning look.

I shrugged.

"I've got another job for you anyway." He held up a computer-printed satellite map and pointed at a red mark that had been made near a road. Apparently there had been a major crew-related find on the other side of the county. "Do you know how to get here?" Shane asked.

At first I didn't recognize the area. It was drawn on such a small scale, that it made the familiar town of Bronson look quite a bit larger than it really was. In fact, it gave me the impression of a town that would have several stoplights, rather than only a handful of stop signs. When it dawned on me that I was looking at a satellite photo of Bronson, I instantly recognized the familiar road. Three of the other recoveries had been made just off that very same road. "That's the other end of Houson Hollow Road, isn't it?"

Shane nodded and answered. "I believe so."

"Sure, I can get there."

While we were talking, Chad Murray and Brother Fred Raney pulled into the parking lot behind us. Shane motioned them over and gave them the details on the newest site. He wanted us to go out to the scene, let Fred conduct the recovery service, then return to Hemphill to pick up the other remains at the sheriff's department sally port.

During the early part of this conversation I was given a somewhat humorous insight into the stress of command. When they first started talking, Chad and Shane misunderstood each other and Chad thought Shane was talking about the site in Six Mile. When Chad realized that Shane was referring to a second site, he said, "Oh, so there's another site." Now it was Shane's turn to misunderstand. He thought Chad didn't know about the Six Mile site. This would mean Brother Raney—whose prayers were a priority of respect with NASA—had missed the first site altogether. Both sites were quickly wrapping up, it would be almost impossible to get Fred to both sites in time, and finding a second chaplain on such short notice would be yet another headache.

"You mean you haven't been out to Six Mile?" Shane asked, suddenly very serious.

"No, we just came from there," Chad replied.

Shane breathed a quick sigh of relief. "I almost wigged out there."

Before we got underway, Shane brought up the question of the Excursion being able to make it down the muddy road. I suggested we come in from the eastern portion of the road so we could miss a notoriously muddy stretch near Bronson. Once again, the scale of the photo threw me. Chad looked at the map and told me this site was very close to Bronson. We would still be well short of the quagmire. He suggested we go up Highway 184 all the way to Bronson and hook around, coming in from the west.

Since I wasn't sure if I could recognize the road coming from that direction, Chad led the way as we pulled out of the parking lot.

* * *

Chad's advice served us well. There's no doubt that after the heavy rain we had early last week, Houson Hollow Road would have been even muddier than it had been on our previous trips if we'd gone the other direction. However, our short trip down the road from the west was relatively easy, with very little slipping and sliding. Still, when we reached the site, the shoulders were far too muddy to park off the road. The FBI rental cars were lined down the center of the road, forcing us to park a good distance from the site.

We pulled in behind another FBI agent who was just arriving. I recognized his face but couldn't tag a name to it. I got the jump cot out of the Excursion and followed the agent up the road.

Up ahead, I saw Terry standing near the edge of the woods, waiting on us.

"I didn't think I'd see you here," the agent ahead of us said. "I thought you were off today."

Terry laughed and shook his head. "I had to make a flying trip to Dallas and back. Not exactly a day off."

Terry shook hands and spoke briefly with each of us before turning and leading the way. The site wasn't far into the woods. After barely a hundred yards I saw a small cluster of FBI agents. I instantly recognized them; it was Debbie's team.

Also present were a pair of ladies from D-Mort, the federal government's disaster mortuary unit. I felt a strange pang of territorialism when I first laid eyes on them. Odd as it may sound, I felt they were stepping in on my job. Then again, although it was only a week into the operation, many of the locals who had started this operation in some position of responsibility had been replaced by a federal expert. Maybe this was our replacement.

At first I thought there wasn't an astronaut present; then I saw two agents and a man in a blue jumpsuit moving in the woods behind me. Before making the recovery, the Evidence Response Team would go over the place with a fine-tooth comb, making sure nothing was left behind. Apparently these two men and this astronaut were making one last sweep of the woods before returning to the site.

The two agents joined us from one direction, but the astronaut came around by another and found his path blocked by dense underbrush. Since I was closest, I tried to help by meeting him halfway. I only ended up getting myself tangled in the briars for my efforts. In fact, the astronaut had to get himself out of the thicket, and then come to my rescue. After pulling me free, the astronaut introduced himself as Jeff Ashby.

Everything at the site was in order and ready to go when we arrived. The photographs had already been taken, and the surrounding area had already been searched. Fred's prayer was all they were waiting on. As soon as Jeff joined us, we made a circle, lowered our heads, and prayed.

Once they finished, the item was carefully placed in a body bag and carried out of the woods on the jump cot.

After loading the cot into the back of the Excursion, Jeff took a moment to thank Terry for all the hard work he and the rest of the agents had put in during this recovery. He said he was particularly impressed with all the courtesy and respect shown to the remains. I think Terry's reply summed up how we all felt about the recovery.

"They're heroes. This is how they should be treated."

* * *

When we returned to Hemphill I backed into the sally port and they shut the gate behind me. The other site hadn't been cleared yet, so we would have to sit tight for a while.

I didn't catch the last name of the agent assigned to remain with the evidence, but her first name was Heidi. She was an intelligent and polite lady—very polite. In fact, when she was accidentally locked out of the sally port, she didn't fuss at the jailor who was manning the gate, or me, who had told him to shut it. She patiently stood outside the gate—since she could see the Excursion, she wasn't violating her duty of remaining with the evidence. After a minute or two we noticed she was locked out; we opened the gate so she could join us.

Kenneth Walton, one of the jailors, joined Jeff, and Heidi and me in the sally port while we waited for the remains to come in from Six Mile. It was a strange little group—Kenneth and me—a pair of native-born country boys, shooting the bull with an FBI agent and an astronaut with four shuttle missions under his belt. We talked about everything from the recovery to the weather before the conversation finally moved on to the space program. Needless to say, Jeff took over from there. He talked about shuttle missions, the space station, the future of NASA, and answered every question we could conjure up. He managed not to go over our heads without once giving us the slightest impression that he was talking down to us. The whole conversation reminded me of those precious few college professors who are so passionate about their field of expertise that their enthusiasm becomes contagious, infecting their audience with extreme interest, leaving them hanging on every word.

About an hour after we arrived, we received word that the Six Mile site had been cleared, and the Humvee was on its way to Hemphill. We opened the sally port so I could pull out and the Humvee could pull in as soon as it arrived. However, no sooner had we opened the gate than a photographer parked across the street started snapping pictures. I pointed her out to Heidi, and she asked Kenneth to close the gate and wait until the Humvee arrived before we opened it.

Thirty minutes later the Humvee pulled in the drive, followed by the big white FBI van. We opened the gate and I pulled out, letting the Humvee pull in. I backed the Excursion in behind it.

Three men got out of the vehicle, two soldiers and an officer. The officer was Captain Mike Kurst. Ironically, Mike was also a funeral director employed at Dorman Funeral Home in Orange.

After the remains were transferred to the Excursion I had time to speak with Mike. I already knew he was in the area. Last Monday I had called Dorman's to ask them for assistance with a graveside service in Orange so Dad and I could stay on call in Hemphill. They had told me that they would love to help, but they couldn't spare anyone since one of their directors was helping out with the National Guard. Mike was curiously apologetic. He had said the way the people of Sabine County had been so nice to the guardsmen, he would certainly do anything he could for someone from this area and hated that they had been unable to help. I had thanked him for the compliment, but told him the apology was unnecessary.

I also had a chance to speak briefly to the leader of the recovery team that had been at the Six Mile site. Earlier, during the trip out to the second site, I did a little thinking about my brief, somewhat less than friendly encounter at the first site of the day. Upon reflection, I realized that the misunderstanding had actually been my fault. Although I was only trying to be helpful, my outburst of suggestions would have seemed like I was telling him how to do his job. If I had been in his shoes, I can't say that I would have reacted any differently.

With this in mind, I waited until he was passing by the Excursion and commented, "Now I see why y'all like those white body bags."

He stopped. "Excuse me?"

"The notes," I said, pointing at the black writing all over the surface of the bag -notes about the position and condition of the body. "You couldn't have written those notes on our black bags."

This time he took the olive branch. He stopped and gave me a brief description of the bags, telling me they're also a lot tougher than they look. Don't get me wrong, we didn't exactly kiss and make up. He was still blunt and somewhat condescending, but, then again, he wasn't here for a popularity contest. Like me, he was here to help return seven heroes to their families, and from all accounts, it was a job he was doing quite well.

* * *

The escorts were gathered and the necessary arrangements for the transportation were made. Jeff would be riding with me. One of the members of the team at Six Mile would be serving as the agent in charge of the evidence, riding along behind us in a rental car. Another pair of agents would follow behind her car, and a DPS patrol car behind them.

We were told that there had also been a crew-related find in San Augustine County. A van would meet us at the intersection of Highways 96 and 103. They would give us another item to transport on to Lufkin.

Right before we left, one of the astronauts approached and asked if I was Squeaky's son. He then asked if I had a lead foot like my father. I laughed and told him I wasn't as bad. They wanted me to lead again, but seventy miles an hour would be plenty. Dad wouldn't hear the end of this one—months later I would still be ribbing him about the fact that his driving had scared professional test pilots.

We pulled out of the driveway and started toward Lufkin at an easy, un-Squeaky-like pace—about sixty-five miles per hour.

* * *

A plain white van belonging to NASA was waiting for us just before we reached the overpass. Jeff got out of the Excursion to speak to the astronauts while I received and loaded a small white cooler.

As soon as the cooler was in place, I joined Jeff and the other astronauts. I had little to add to the conversation, but I was certainly flattered to be among them—even more so when Jeff politely introduced me to the other two astronauts. During the brief roadside conversation, Jeff told one of the astronauts there was only one more crewmember to go.

When we got back into the Excursion, I told Jeff that I knew we were getting close, but I had no idea that today's find put us one discovery away from our goal. He said that when this operation began he never would have imagined that we would have such success in such a short period of time. It was very possible that tomorrow we would find the last of the seven, completing the most important portion of the operation in only eleven days.

I was also hopeful, but I had one nagging doubt in my mind. The search teams had almost walked the entire length of the county, and they were coming up on the lake. In fact, the lake was only a mile from where the last discovery had been made. What if the last body was in the lake?

However, I didn't state my doubts to Jeff, and by the time we reached Lufkin I was fully infected by his good humor and enthusiasm. I just knew tomorrow would be the day we would find the seventh astronaut.

26
The Red Cross

JANIE JOHNSON WOKE around 4:30 AM to start the drive to Sabine County. As Service Delivery Manager of the Red Cross's Orange Chapter—which also covers Orange, Newton, Sabine, San Augustine, Angelina and Nacogdoches Counties—she needed to be back in Hemphill as soon as possible. The day before had not been a good one. While on an important business trip to Baltimore, she had often found her thoughts wandering to the recovery effort in Texas. It had taken several frustrating hours to get back to East Texas, including almost getting snowed in at Baltimore and getting stuck in a major traffic jam in Houston. While sitting in her car waiting for the stalled traffic to inch forward, Janie received three pages wanting to know where she was and how soon she could leave for Hemphill. These pages added to her frustration, as well as her determination to get back to where she was needed.

Janie finally arrived in Orange at around seven o'clock. She washed her clothes, packed her bags, and then settled in for some much-needed sleep. At five-thirty in the morning she was on the road for Hemphill.

Her instructions were to find her supervisor, Bob Martin, get briefed on the current situation, and relieve him. Coming up Highway 87 she turned off on the highway that would lead her to the VFW and fair grounds. As her truck made the curve her mouth dropped and she had to pull off to the side of the road. She had never seen so many DPS cars, military trucks, and people in one place. They were everywhere. It seemed like a lifetime since she left Hemphill on the second evening of the recovery effort, and it certainly seemed as if a lifetime's worth of changes had taken place.

After finding a parking place, Janie proceeded to the storeroom. The Red Cross volunteers were currently working out of the VFW kitchen, helping Belinda Gay's local group of cooks. The VFW hall's back meeting room had been converted into a multipurpose storage room. Some of the items "stored" in the room were the Red Cross volunteers who slept on cots aligned along the walls. Janie, thinking how tired they all looked, received hugs from each volunteer and they all started telling her what had happened since she left last week. It felt good to be back. Now, she needed to find Bob and relieve him so he could go home and get some rest.

When she finally found Bob, he looked as though he had not slept in a week. He told her about all that had changed and gave her a detailed description of the daily schedule. After the briefing, they started toward town. Janie had a lot of new faces to learn.

The first stop was the National Guard Command at the Sabine County Rodeo Arena—while the majority of the troops' quarters were at the Hemphill High School, their command and most of their equipment and supplies were out at the rodeo arena. The National Guard had proved to be a great asset to the operation. Not only were they one of the most efficient search groups in the field, but their support personnel always went out of their way to assist any other group or organization in need. This two-way street was one of the greatest aspects of the operation, and the link between the National Guard and the Red Cross served as a fine example of the smooth links that were established between the majority of the organizations involved. If the National Guard needed anything, the Red Cross would do anything they could to help, and if the Red Cross needed anything, the National Guard would do the same. If Janie needed something moved that was too heavy for her crew, if they needed a few extra hands at the VFW hall, or if everyone was busy and they simply needed someone to make a supply run, the National Guard would find a way to get the job done.

Later that night, Janie would pay an interesting visit to National Guard Command. One of the Red Cross's many responsibilities was to serve as a link between soldiers performing their duties and their families back home. Earlier in the night, the Red Cross had received a routine request from a concerned family member; so shortly after nightfall, Janie made her way up to the rodeo arena to perform a health and welfare check. She imagined that many of the soldiers were already asleep, so she opened the door as slowly and quietly as possible. Inside the command she found the twenty or so soldiers who were stationed there fast asleep, except for the one guard on duty. The sound of so many people snoring from heavy sleep made the place sound like a jungle. Not a single night owl could be found among the camouflage and olive drab gear and bedding; they were exhausted from the day's work. It was strangely humorous and touching at the same time. Janie took care of the inquiry by speaking with the guard on duty. Sleep was a precious thing to these hardworking soldiers and it would be better if she didn't have to wake the soldier in question.

The next stop was the Incident Command Post. The fire hall was hardly recognizable from her last visit. There was an officer stationed at the outside of the door and another behind a sign-in table on the inside. On the inside, dividers now separated the hall into several small offices, and there were about ten times the number of people present as there had been a week ago. As they made their way through the crowd, Bob introduced Janie to several new faces and reacquainted her with the people she had met the previous week. She spoke with the people directly over her in the chain of command, Incident Commanders Sheriff Maddox and Billy Ted Smith, as well as Logistics Chief Mark Allan. She also spoke with Marcus Beard, a name she easily remembered due to word association—Marcus was sporting a short, heavy beard. She also touched base with the hardworking FBI duo of Shane Ball and Terry Lane. She had only met them a little over a week ago, yet returning to the Command Post was like getting to see old friends again.

Bob gave Janie a map and names so she could finish making the rounds while he started home for some much needed rest. The next stop on Janie's list was twenty miles south of Hemphill, in the small community of Fairmount. The Navy divers had recently set up their command post at the Fairmount Volunteer Fire Department's fire hall. Since their new post was quite a distance away from the VFW Hall, the Red Cross would be taking their meals out to them. Janie spoke with the FEMA officer at the Fairmount fire hall, writing down all the information needed to see that their needs were met.

Since the Fairmount fire hall was a new post, the meeting with the FEMA officer took quite some time. It was several hours before Janie returned to the VFW hall and helped Belinda Gay plan for the next day. Janie couldn't help but be impressed with Belinda and her hard working crew at the VFW hall.

After meeting with Belinda, Janie rounded up a pair of her volunteers. They took two trucks to Jasper for supplies. The trio of volunteers was exhausted from the long day; this made the two hour trip seem to last forever. When they returned, the volunteers unloaded and stored the supplies. It was around midnight before the Red Cross volunteers retired to their cots on the empty end of the storage area.

* * *

A typical day for the Red Cross volunteers began long before the first of the search volunteers arrived at the VFW Post. Not long after the VFW cooks began preparing breakfasts, the Red Cross volunteers would climb out of their cots to begin serving the meal. Once the search volunteers arrived, they found the long buffet line and drink table manned by the cooks who had finished their duties in the kitchen and Red Cross volunteers.

Once the searchers had moved from breakfast to morning preparations, the volunteers began cleaning the VFW Post's hall and kitchen area. This was truly a group effort, as volunteers from the kitchen, the local high schools, the Red Cross, and several unaffiliated walk-on volunteers pitched in to tidy up the place.

The next order of the day was to help prepare the meals that would be taken out to the searchers in the field. Once the sack lunches were prepared, the Red Cross volunteers were responsible for seeing that the meals made it to their destination. The National Guard was self-sufficient in this regard; in order to cut down on the logistics of feeding so many searchers in the field, they relied on the rations they took with them. However, this still left several hundred hungry workers and volunteers to be fed. Hundreds of meals were piled into the Orange Red Cross Chapter's Emergency Response Vehicle, a large equipment truck nicknamed "Big Red." These meals were then taken to the day's planned mid-day break area.

Once the Red Cross workers returned to the VFW Hall they helped prepare for the afternoon meal. They pitched in with various other organizations and individual volunteers to prepare and serve a massive meal.

At the end of the day, the Red Cross volunteers were often used to bring in supplies. They were often still pushing carts, loading and unloading groceries well after dark.

The best type of volunteer for any operation is the person who arrives as soon as possible and gladly takes their place wherever they are needed. In this regard, the Red Cross volunteers typify the majority of the volunteers in this operation.

27
The Last of the Seven Heroes

TUESDAY'S CALL CAME at about one o'clock, much earlier than normal. When I arrived at the Sheriff's Department, I could feel the excitement. A man in an FBI jacket directed me to back up to the sally port where a Humvee was already waiting.

I opened the door, but before I even got out of the driver's seat I asked a DPS officer who was standing nearby, "Do we have the last one?"

"I think so," he replied with a smile.

I assisted in loading the body bag onto the jump cot and placing it in the back of the Excursion. After I was finished, an astronaut whose face was very familiar but whose name I had yet to catch, asked if I would mind making the run straight to Barksdale Air Force Base. I told them I would be honored. Although I did know where the base was located, I didn't know where to go once I got to the base. Dad had told me that in order to avoid the media, the funeral home that had been transporting the astronauts from Lufkin to Barksdale hadn't been using the main gate. I wasn't sure where this secondary entrance was located.

The astronaut told me not to worry about finding the gate. He would find someone to lead me there.

While the astronauts returned to the command center to arrange for the transportation, I went inside the sheriff's office and called Caraway Funeral Home. I spoke with Roy Caraway, and asked him if there was anything in particular that I needed to know about the run to Barksdale. He told me that I needed to phone in before I reached the base so they would be ready for me when I got there.

When I went back outside, Michael was still across the road at the ICP. However, he had already arranged for a Texas DPS escort at least as far as the state line; these two officers' patrol pickup was already parked in front of the Sheriff's Department. I spoke to them and they told me that they would lead me all the way if they needed to, and that they knew how to get to Barksdale.

After speaking briefly with the officers, I recognized one of the FBI agents parked in a nearby SUV. Although he had served as my escort on several occasions and he was certainly one of the agents I knew and recognized, I never did get his name. He was a little older than most of the agents I had dealt with, and his shirt identified him as an FBI firearms instructor.

Although I didn't know this agent's name, he was quick to help me out on the name of the astronaut in charge. Michael Lopez-Alegria had been very active throughout the recovery, but, unlike the other astronauts, I couldn't simply look at his nametag and tell who he was. At this point all I knew was that I had overheard someone calling him Michael "Something-or-other," but his nametag really threw me for a curve. It simply read, "L.-A.". I not only discovered that he really did have a last name, but I found out he was an astronaut with ten years' experience, who had served on three different shuttle missions, including performing a pair of spacewalks on his second mission, STS-92 Discovery, in October of 2000.

We were still talking about Michael when he returned from the command center to give us an update. He said we would definitely be taking the remains on to Barksdale. He just had to make a few more phone calls to make sure everybody along the chain of command was aware of this little change in procedure.

After Michael started back across the road to the command center, I noticed something about the Excursion—it was filthy. Over the last couple of weeks, the trusty old SUV had seen its share of muddy roads. Currently, there was more brown mud showing than black paint.

I went back into the sheriff's office and found Sheriff Maddox. "Can I ask a favor?"

"Sure," he said at first. Then he thought better of it, smiled, and said, "Well, it depends. What's the favor?"

"They're talking about sending me straight to Barksdale and the Excursion is a mess. Can I get a couple of the trustees to give it a quick wash-job?"

"No problem."

"Maybe they should just rinse it off," I added. "I don't know how long we have. I'm sure they'll want us to roll as soon as they get permission."

Tom said he imagined we would have more than enough time, and, as it turned out, he was right. In fact, the trustees were able to give the DPS pickup that would be serving as my escort a quick cleaning as well.

Less than thirty minutes later, while the trustees were just beginning to rinse the soap off the pickup, I saw Michael returning from the command center.

From here on out, everything happened fast, almost with a sense of urgency. The two DPS patrol officers, the FBI firearms instructor, Michael, the new astronaut, and I gathered in the parking lot, near the edge of the road. The DPS officers would escort us to the state line where a Louisiana State Trooper would take over, leading us on to Barksdale. The FBI agent would follow behind us, serving as Evidence Officer.

After some brief instructions, we climbed into our vehicles and Michael returned to the command center. I noticed that the astronaut got into the car with the FBI agent and wondered if I should mention that the ride-along astronaut usually rode with me. I hadn't seen this particular astronaut before, maybe he didn't know. However, everything happened so fast. We were in the cars and pulling off before we knew it, the trustees rinsing the patrol pickup even as it pulled away.

While I felt unworthy of the position, I was flattered at

the opportunity to serve as both driver and impromptu honor guard.

* * *

We missed our Louisiana escort at the Texas/Louisiana border, so the two DPS officers escorted us the whole way in. Thank God for Michael's foresight in seeing that the escorts knew how to get to the back entrance at Barksdale, even though they weren't supposed to lead us the entire way.

We pulled up at a gate that was across a wide field from the buildings that marked the main portion of the base. A concrete barrier was positioned in the road so that a car entering the gate would have to slow down in order to proceed. I wondered briefly if this barrier had been present before September 11, 2001. Overhead, B-52s were circling in and landing on the short runway located in the middle of the field—a grim reminder of the coming war with Iraq.

When we arrived at the gate, only one soldier was at the post. I waited in the car while he spoke to the astronaut. The guard allowed us in, but we stopped just inside the gate to wait for an escort to come and lead us to our destination.

I got out and joined the rest of our group and the guard at the hood of the Excursion. We talked about the recovery and about Iraq, while watching the massive war machines soaring overhead.

The B-52s' engines screamed at such a volume that we were forced to cover our ears every time they came in. I had already counted well over a dozen that had landed and could see three more circling. I was about to ask how many there were and how they could land on such a short runway when I noticed something—there were actually only four B-52s in the air; they were practicing taking off and landing by touching down, lifting back off, and then circling around for another go. I felt like a real idiot but I figured we could all use a good laugh, even if it was at my expense, so I told the group about my little mistake. My confession immediately set off a barrage of *You Think That's Bad* stories that helped pass the time.

We didn't have to wait long for our escort to arrive. After a few minutes, the guard received a call on his radio. The base escort was on the way. Sure enough, barely a minute passed before a white patrol car with Barksdale Air Force Base stenciled on the side pulled up. The driver motioned for us to follow him.

* * *

We pulled through the high cyclone fences topped with barbwire and continued past the armed guards. As we slowly drove among the massive hangars I saw that while my earlier misconception that dozens of B-52s were landing might have been incorrect, there were certainly enough bombers here to make that mistake a reality. There were B-52s everywhere, over two dozen in the immediate area, and that includes only those in plain sight—there could have been any number tucked away in the massive hangars.

Our escort led us around one of the closed hangars and into a small parking lot that was almost empty. There was a pair of swinging doors on the side of the hangar, much too small for a B-52, but extremely large doors nonetheless. An Air Force sergeant walked out into the parking lot to meet us. He motioned for my three escort vehicles to park off to the side and directed me to back up to the small rectangular bier positioned about fifty feet in front of the wide hangar doors.

It wasn't until I stopped and got out of the Excursion that I got a good look at what was waiting at the doors of the hangar. A full military honor guard was standing at attention, lined on either side of the open hangar doors. A second, larger bier was positioned just inside, flanked by an American and an Israeli flag. Two chaplains and an officer stood near the bier. No crowds were present, no politicians, and certainly no press. Just like the prayers Brother Raney had said back in the piney woods of East

Texas, this wasn't for show. This was an homage to one of the seven fallen heroes.

The sergeant asked me to open the back doors of the Excursion. I did, then I climbed into the back of the Excursion as I had done so often while making recoveries over the last couple of days. I knew the jump cot's front wheels would often get caught in the wells made for the SUV's back seat. The honor guard could have managed without my assistance, but I guess it was the funeral director in me that made me climb into the back of the Excursion. I wanted to make sure everything went off smoothly.

The main portion of the honor guard remained at attention, while the pallbearers approached in perfect unison. The first two reached inside and grasped the cot, and I helped by lifting from my end as they pulled it out, making sure the wheels didn't get stuck.

As soon as the jump cot left my hands, I was struck by the magnificence of what I was witnessing. I was overwhelmed. My eyes grew misty as the pallbearers slowly returned to the hangar with the last astronaut between them.

When they entered the hangar and set the cot on the bier, I recalled something I had told my father after the first day of recoveries. I told him that when it was all said and done, I wanted to know whom we had recovered. I wanted to be able to put a name and a face to the two heroes we had helped return home that day. I now realized that this feeling no longer troubled me. I could easily place names and faces to those we had helped, because we had been part of all seven recoveries.

And now the last of those seven heroes was going home.

I remained cramped in the back of the Excursion during the entire ceremony, watching the scene as it unfolded before me, framed by the Excursion's open back doors. It was as if I was afraid to climb out, afraid that the sound of my shoes touching the pavement would break the precious silence. From where I sat, the words of prayer were distant whispers—I couldn't make out a single word. Once the prayers were said, the hangar doors were slowly pulled shut.

28

The Memorial Service and Beyond

THERE WERE MANY MEMORIALS given for the crewmembers of STS-107 Columbia throughout the days following their tragic death. However, the operation's personnel were unable to attend any of these services. In fact, since they were working from sunup to sundown, they usually missed the services that were aired from Houston, Washington, and all over the United States and Israel.

The idea to hold a memorial service in Hemphill was brought up in a conversation between Greg Cohrs and Astronaut Brent Jett even before I left for Barksdale AFB with the last crewmember. The one-mile search corridor through the heart of Sabine County would be completed by Thursday evening. There was still much work to be done, as the area would have to be gone over again to make sure nothing had been missed, and the search corridor would be widened in order to search for items outside of the initial one-mile corridor. However, it was decided that once the main corridor was completed, the search effort would be suspended for one day so the people participating in the Sabine County recovery effort could attend the service.

Like the search effort itself, the memorial service was a group effort. Several local commanders and astronauts who had worked in the county were to speak at the service. Belinda Gay and the kitchen team at the VFW post saw to the initial preparations. Mary Beth Gray, owner of Hemphill Flower Shop, prepared seven wreaths, one for each of the crewmembers. The local elementary schools even played a part. Since Friday was

Valentine's Day, the children colored and cut out red and purple hearts to decorate the walls.

The search continued on Wednesday and Thursday. Spirits were high on the line and at the ICP, and several pieces of debris were located and recovered. The most important part of the operation was already a success, but there was still a lot of work to be done.

The memorial was scheduled for eight o'clock Friday morning, but many of the volunteers arrived early. Over the last couple of weeks they had grown accustomed to rising early and getting to the VFW post before sunrise. The veterans took their customary seats among familiar search team members and search team leaders.

The service began when each of the seven wreaths was escorted down the center isle in the VFW hall. Once all the wreaths were in place, the speakers took their turns at the podium. The two original co-commanders spoke briefly, as did many representatives of the various organizations and volunteer groups. The pinnacle of the service, however, was Brent Jett's eulogy. He presented us with a look into the astronauts we had worked so hard to see were returned home to their families. His eulogy was a personal touch that was greatly appreciated by everyone present.

* * *

Despite having recovered all seven astronauts, successfully completing the primary goal of the operation, there was still much work to be done. The shuttle recovery operation would continue for several months, growing into the largest ground search in United States history.

Following the memorial service, the recovery efforts in Sabine and San Augustine Counties were merged under the direction of one of the National Incident Management Teams. The Incident Command Post for the continuing search was relocated to the Sabine County VFW Hall and Fairgrounds. "Camp Hemphill" was established for the 1500-1700 national firefighters, NASA and EPA personnel, and other incident personnel that would continue the search and recovery efforts in an effort to determine the cause of the tragedy. The Hemphill post was one of four, the others being in Nacogdoches, Palestine, and Corsicana. Camp Hemphill ceased operations on April 22nd.

While most of the volunteers were sent home after the second week, this did not mark the end of the local involvement in the search efforts. Many of the same people who had been there in the beginning would still play important roles in the command system. While the operation became largely self-sufficient, it still relied on local ambulance crews and other local emergency assets as a backup for their own emergency medical system. Likewise, local law enforcement still played an important role as security for the operation. Also, since the U.S. Forest Service played such a crucial role in the early portion of the recovery, it was only natural that local Forest Service employees would remain directly involved. One duty that fell on their shoulders was assisting in orientating and organizing the new search teams that would be arriving in the area. Greg Cohrs continued to serve as a Branch Director for 400-600 searchers and other Sabine and Angelina National Forest employees continued to lead search teams.

* * *

I can think of no better symbolic tribute to the operation than the fact that the Incident Command Post and the Volunteer Staging Area in Sabine County were located at the Hemphill Volunteer Fire Department's fire hall and the local Veterans of Foreign Wars post. Long before the wave of volunteerism washed over the county on February 1, 2003, the county's firefighters had been volunteers for their fellow man. Likewise, our veterans had answered their country's call long before this newest call for help.

There are those who say the people of Sabine County have changed since Columbia fell into our midst. The people haven't changed; it just took this tragedy to allow the world to see how helpful, hard-working and caring the people of this community are. The people who waded into the thickest underbrush and the coldest creeks, working long, hard days, were the same people who braved fires to help save their neighbor's lives and property. The same hands that prepared food for the searchers and the workers had often prepared food for the sick and bereaved. The police officers who worked on the response teams were on duty protecting their neighbors long before the shuttle went down; the federal employees and incident leaders trained and prepared to handle disasters and served in other disaster efforts long before they were called into action to recover Columbia's heroes.

What happened in Sabine County—and other communities along Columbia's corridor—serves as a good microcosm for our great nation. On the surface, America has changed since 9/11, but the people are the same. We were always there, and we were always proud of our country. The response to the tragedy brought out the best in the community as they served their nation, and the world had the opportunity to see how great the people of rural East Texas really are.

* * *

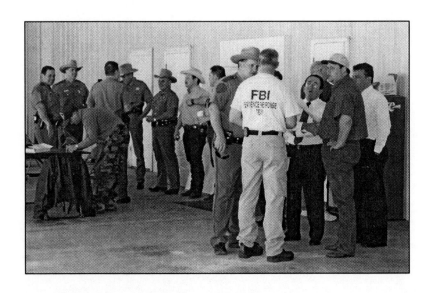

Pictures from the author's collection:

"In the right side of this photo is a group of five men in a circle, just prior to going out to the first site. The circle, from left to right: DPS Sergeant Tommy Scales, Terry Lane of the FBI (his back is to us), John Starr Jr. (my father), Chief Deputy Chad Murray, and me."

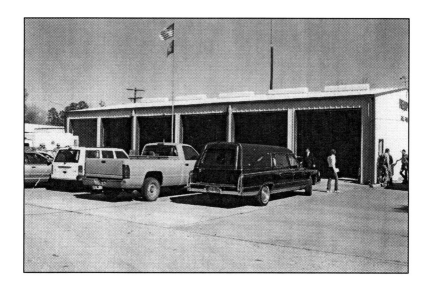

Pictures from the author's collection:

Prior to going to the first site. The author, in suit and tie, stands in front of the hearse.

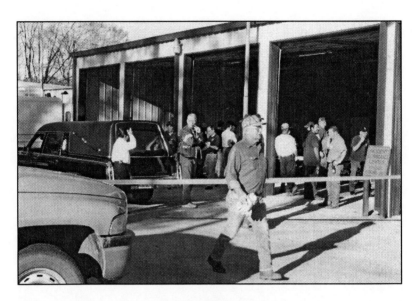

Pictures from the author's collection:

"This is after our return from the first scene; in fact, at this point I'm still out at the first scene. Behind the hearse is my father, John Starr Jr., and Brother Fred Raney. D.B. Chance (Hemphill's Fire Chief) is in the foreground and the man in the fourth bay from the left with a radio on his hip, talking on the cell phone, is Hemphill City Manager Don Iles. The tall man behind him is Bob Morgan (Six Mile Fire Chief)."

About the Author

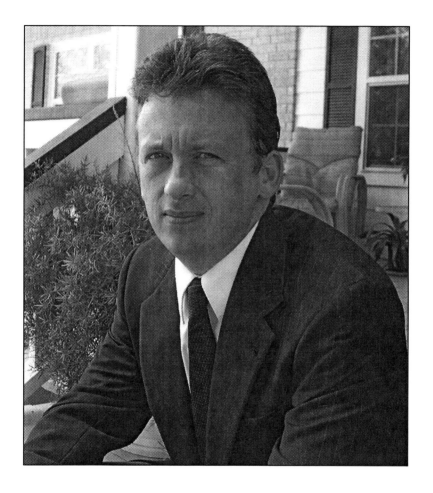

In 1992 Byron attended the Dallas Institute of Funeral Service and the following year he served his funeral directing and embalming apprenticeship under his father. In 1993 he married Shelly Rolfe. It wasn't until the autumn of 1999 that his reading hobby branched into a writing hobby.

Other Titles from Liaison Press:

The Mask of Oyá, by Flor Fernández Barrios. (Memoir/
Spirituality, ISBN 189495338X, SRP $14.95):
Flor Fernández Barrios shares her experiences in transforming
herself from an awkward, anxious girl, recently immigrated from
Cuba, into a confident curandera healer, following the wisdom
of her grandmother and embracing her culture. From the author
of *Blessed by Thunder,* this is a voyage you won't soon forget.

*You're Not Very Important: 12 Steps Away from Self-esteem and Toward
a Better World,* by Douglas W. Texter. (Satire/Self-help, ISBN
1894953207, SRP $13.95 US):
Almost-Dr. Douglas Texter takes his readers on a whirlwind tour
of the practice of self-betterment throughout the ages in this
biting parody of self-help literature. He carefully explores the
Big 12 myths of self-improvement, and at the same time, delivers
a devastating, sardonic social and political commentary.

Random Acts of Malice: The Best of Happy Woman Magazine
edited by Sharon Grehan. (Parody/Satire, ISBN 1894953320,
SRP $13.95 US):
Random Acts of Malice features a selection of the wickedest
(and funniest) articles from the last five years of *Happy Woman
Magazine.* Featuring work by some of the best satirists on the
planet: Sharon Grehan, Elizabeth Hanes, Elaine Langlois,
Pamela Monk, Jessica Becht, Mike Boone, Crystal Click,
Christina Delia, Stephen James, Meredith Litt, Susan Shoemaker,
Diane Sokoloski, Sarah Szucs, and Julie Ward...Can you afford
NOT to buy this book?

Printed in the United States
69926LV00003B/7-45